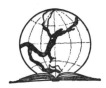

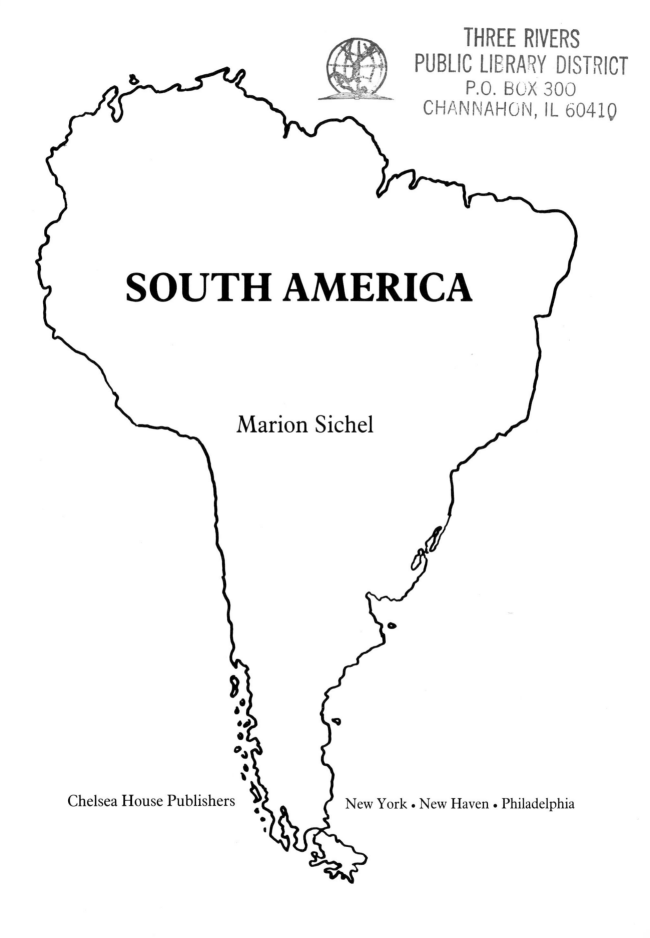

SOUTH AMERICA

Marion Sichel

Chelsea House Publishers   New York • New Haven • Philadelphia

Printed in Great Britain

Published in the U.S.A. by
Chelsea House Publishers
5014 West Chester Pike
Edgemont, Pa., 19028

Published in the U.K. by
B T Batsford Limited
4 Fitzhardinge Street,
London W1H 0AH

Library of Congress Cataloging in Publication Data

Sichel, Marion.
  South America.

  Bibliography: p.
  Summary: Presents in text and illustrations the traditional
costumes of the countries of South America. Includes a full
description of each costume, its cultural significance, its
historical derivation, and the context in which the costume
was worn.
  1. Costume—South America. [1. Costume—South
America] I. Title.
  GT675.S53 1986   391'.0098   86-9730
  ISBN 1-55546-158-1

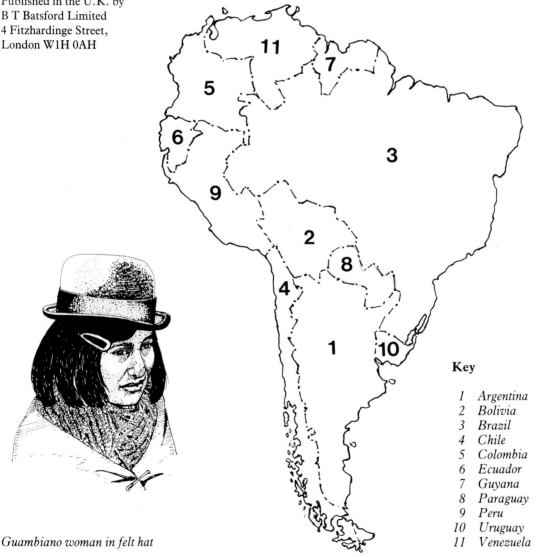

Guambiano woman in felt hat

Key

1   Argentina
2   Bolivia
3   Brazil
4   Chile
5   Colombia
6   Ecuador
7   Guyana
8   Paraguay
9   Peru
10 Uruguay
11 Venezuela

CONTENTS

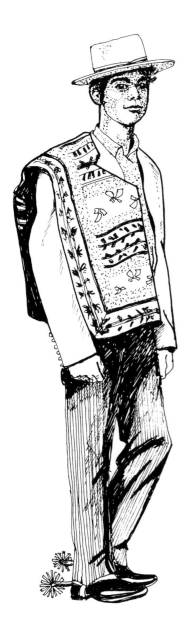

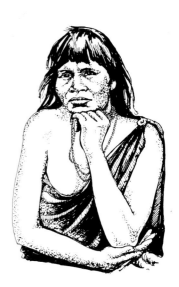

An aboriginal Indian woman from Venezuela in everyday dress of short lengths of coarse material

◄ *Huaso wearing a broad brimmed felt hat and a short multi-coloured poncho over a white shirt. Large silver spurs are worn*

PREFACE

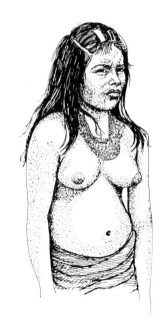

Many of the traditional costumes of the South American countries are no longer seen or are disappearing fast as industrialisation and modern technology encroach on hitherto inaccessible areas.

The traditional dress described and illustrated in this book is typical of national and regional styles still being worn today in areas which, so far, have been least affected by modern civilisation, but many are now worn purely on festive occasions or merely as tourist attractions.

As far more information can be conveyed by drawings than by words, the text is kept to the minimum concentrating on the context in which the costumes can be seen; the climatic and environmental aspects affecting the type of dress – or lack of it – worn.

It is hoped that the impact of the excellent line drawings will convey the 'flavour' of the traditional costumes of the individual countries and of South America as a whole and inspire the reader to further study.

Girl of the Waunana tribe in Colombia

My most grateful thanks must go to the staff of Canning House Library and the Cultural Liaison Officers of the South American countries who most willingly gave their time to supply information and material for inclusion in the book.

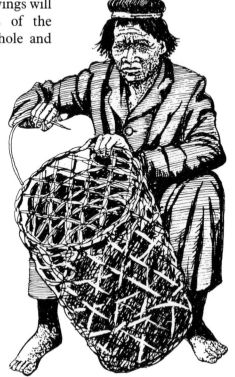

In the remote Indian Amazon villages basket-work is the traditional livelihood

4

INTRODUCTION

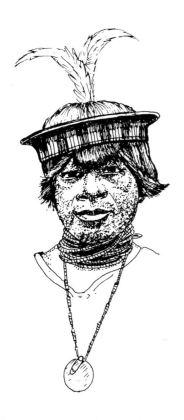

Vaqueiro of the north-east of Brazil wearing a large straw hat

Campa Indian of the Peruvian Montaña known as a Chucupiari, meaning maker of arrows

The New World, by which both North and South America are still known, was not discovered until the end of the fifteenth century. South America was then under Spanish domination for three centuries but as the Spaniards appeared to be interested only in the exploitation of the countries' mineral wealth, mainly gold, development was slow until the beginning of the nineteenth century.

Now, in many parts of South America, industrialisation is on the increase. Modern transportation and communication have opened up previously isolated areas where the wearing of traditional dress was once a natural everyday event, and where now western clothes have taken over. Unfortunately much documentation is so vague that many tribal traditions and dress have been sadly lost. South America, however, is very large, and vast regions still remain unexplored, no doubt concealing treasures to be discovered by future generations.

The evolution of the character and style of the South American national costume is reflected by the pressures of the Spanish and Portuguese colonisation in the sixteenth century, which resulted in widespread interbreeding between these settlers and the indigenous peoples.

Primitive tribes, however, have survived in isolated areas of the various South American countries as well as in many parts of the jungle and forests of the Amazon. The isolation in which they live leaves them relatively untouched by civilisation, some wearing perhaps only coloured beads or feathers in a variety of ways. The performance of their rites and ceremonies characterised by painting their faces and bodies, and for some, nudity is considered a condition of their religious belief and they will only enter the sacred places in the jungle if they are naked. The wearing of ornaments in the form of necklaces, bracelets, headdresses and masks has magical and legendary significance, each object having its own special meaning and each and every tribe having some special form of identity.

In the many countries of South America there is none more popular or more legendary a figure than the 'cowboy': the 'gauchos' of Paraguay and Uruguay, the 'huasos' of Chile, the 'llaneros' of Colombia and the 'vaqueiros' of north-east Brazil. These are the picturesque characters, the riders of the vast pampas plains who have captured the imagination of people worldwide.

From a study of such costumes can be determined the geography, history and industry, as well as religion, education, politics and social aspects of the areas and peoples of the countries in which they originated.

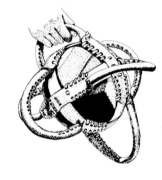

A game of pato played by the gauchos on horseback. Pato *means duck. When this game was originally played a real duck was used, covered in cow hide. This has been replaced by a ball with six handles, and the object of the game is to throw the ball into a big net at the opponents' end of the field*

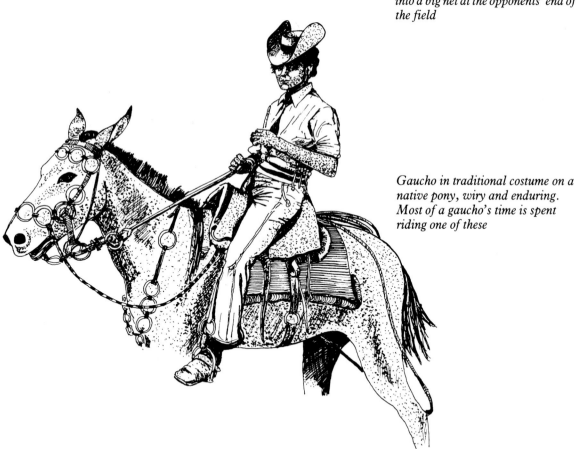

Gaucho in traditional costume on a native pony, wiry and enduring. Most of a gaucho's time is spent riding one of these

6

ARGENTINA

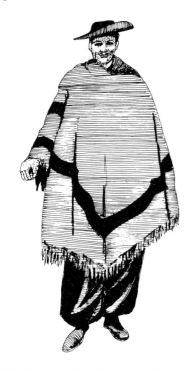

Gaucho wearing a wide poncho, playing his favourite instrument, the guitar

Gaucho wearing a large poncho which can also be used as a blanket

Argentina is a large country, the eighth largest in the world and the second largest in area in South America. A country five times the area of France, Argentina borders Chile to the west. Separated by the Andes, Bolivia and Paraquay are her northern neighbours. Brazil is to the north east; Uruquay to the east. Argentina's geography is not only vast but multi-faceted. The Andes dominate the character of the entire west of the country. In the north and Mesopotamia are the forest plains of the Chaco region. The rich, fertile Pampas region stretches for hundreds of kilometres. Patagonia, in the south, is an inhospitable wind-swept plateau area.

Argentina was not an important part of the Spanish-American empire. Disappointingly, there were few precious metals to be found even though 'arentina' is the Spanish word for 'silver'. Nor was there an abundant labour force in the indigenous Indian people who, far from friendly to the Spanish, were few in number and constantly on the move. Argentina's great wealth lay, as it continues to lie, in her vast resources of rich soils. Buenos Aires, the misnamed 'Good Air', was a further resource as a great port into which the riches of the region could flow.

From the mixture of Spanish and Indians came the famous *gauchos* who for two centuries were to Argentina what the cowboys are to the Western Frontier of the USA.

After Independence in the early nineteenth century, Argentina entered a period of conflict between competing groups. Juan Manuel de Rosas emerged from the turmoil establishing his control by force over the whole country. Rosas was described as having 'applied the knife of the gaucho to the culture of Buenos Aires and destroyed the work of centuries of civilization, law, and liberty'. Rosas in his turn was overthrown after which Argentina enjoyed relative peace and stability before entering a period of remarkable prosperity based upon the exploitation of her agricultural resources. To make this possible as war against the Indians of the Pampas from 1878-83,

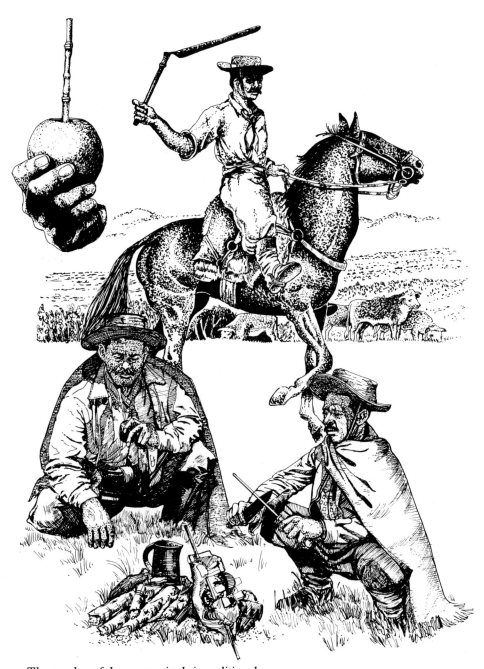

The gauchos of the pampas in their traditional clothes with ponchos and straw hats eating their usual meal of grilled beef and drinking maté, a herbal infusion of leaves that can be drunk hot or cold. Inset is a maté, *which is a recepticle of the same name from which it is drunk*

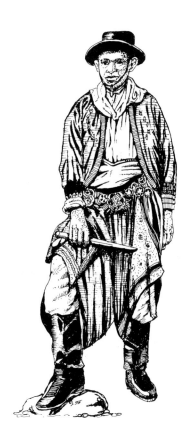

which virtually exterminated them, was necessary. Argentine meat and grain were shipped to Europe, European ideas tastes and fashions entered Argentina. This European impact was dramatic, affecting the entire cultural and political life of the country as well as the economy. For many the prosperity seemed uncheckable. Alas, it was not to be. Firmly caught up in world trade Argentina's prosperity would, henceforth, reflect the ups and downs of other peoples' prosperity. Exports varied dramatically in the first decades of the twentieth century to plummet during the Great Depression of the 1930s. After this time Argentina was forced to rely more upon its own resources and strengths, giving rise to a period of strong nationalistic sentiment.

As the herds of cattle no longer roam wild over the Pampas, the gaucho has become merely a memory, the costume remaining just a traditional dress worn on festive occasions.

The gaucho costume, however, is striking, consisting of a large *poncho*, which is an oblong piece of woollen or alpaca cloth with a slit in the centre for the head to protrude, allowing the folds to cover the shoulders and arms to the elbows, and to fall down in front and behind. Baggy trousers, called *bombachas*, are tucked into high boots made of soft leather to which are attached large silver spurs. Around his waist he wears a belt, often of solid silver into which is tucked a *chirpá*, a square of coloured cloth, which forms a kind of apron. A hat of felt or straw, tied under the chin, is characteristic headgear.

The guacho used, with great skill, the *bolas* which is made up of small stone weights attached to two or three short strong cords that in turn are fastened to a lasso. This is thrown against the legs of running animals to bring them down and thus capture them.

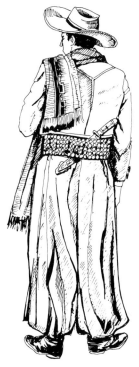

▲
Gaucho wearing long soft leather boots into which his baggy trousers are tucked. Around his waist he wears a solid silver belt which supports the chirpá, *a square of material which forms a kind of apron, and he holds a stiletto in his hand*

◀ *Gaucho wearing baggy trousers called* bombachas, *a shirt and a jacket (usually with silver buttons), a neckerchief and a poncho which can be draped over one shoulder. The wide belt is covered entirely with silver coins. He is also carrying a knife stuck into his belt. The hat is of felt*

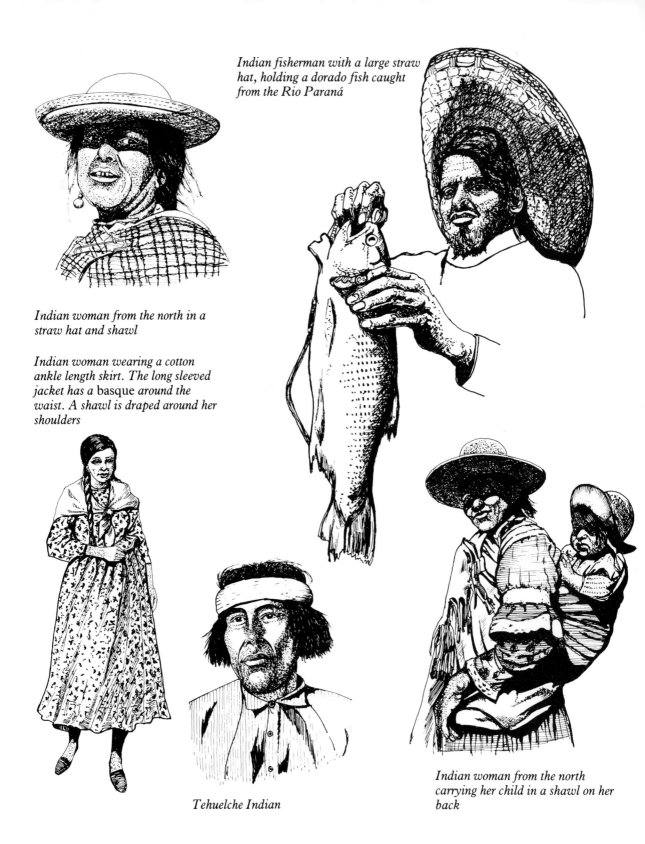

Indian fisherman with a large straw hat, holding a dorado fish caught from the Rio Paraná

Indian woman from the north in a straw hat and shawl

Indian woman wearing a cotton ankle length skirt. The long sleeved jacket has a basque *around the waist. A shawl is draped around her shoulders*

Tehuelche Indian

Indian woman from the north carrying her child in a shawl on her back

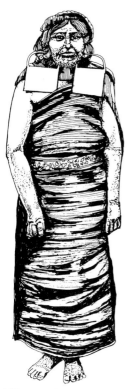

Typical Patagonian woman wearing enormous silver earrings

Patagonia was inhabited by some of the most primitive Indians, known as *Patagonies* or *Big Feet*. There now remain only the Tehuelche Indians who live mostly in the east, which is under the jurisdiction of Argentina. These people are amongst the tallest in the world and are expert hunters and swimmers. It is fashionable for the men to remove all hair from their faces, sometimes even their eyebrows.

The guanaco, a ruminant of the llama family, is one of their most prized possessions, from its wool they weave cloth; they use its skin to make warm outer garments; and from its hide they make their boots and shoes. They wear ornaments of silver, as well as of shells and bone.

The Ona Indians who live in the archipelago of **Tierra del Fuego** are kinsmen of the Tehuelche tribe. Due to the climatic conditions of these parts they dress warmly in guanaco skins in the cold wet winter, and in the short hot summer they go about completely naked. They use bows and arrows to hunt their quarry, and paint their faces with natural dyes. They live the life of true nomads, but are a fast dying race.

The native Yahgan Indians of Tierra del Fuego spend much of their time in canoes or crouched by their fires. They used to wear cloaks of seal skin or otter furs, but with the arrival of the white man, they have been introduced to woollen shawls, blankets and many western garments. Their ornamentation is mainly of shells and bones.

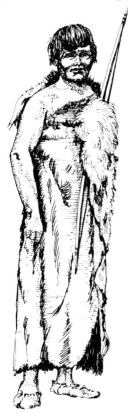

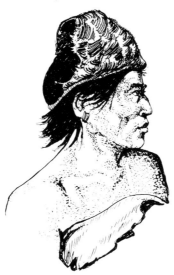

Ona hunter from Tierra del Fuego wearing a fur hat

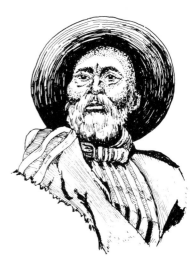

Patagonian Indian in a wide brimmed hat

◀ *An Ona Indian wrapped in a cloak of seal skin under which he might not wear anything*

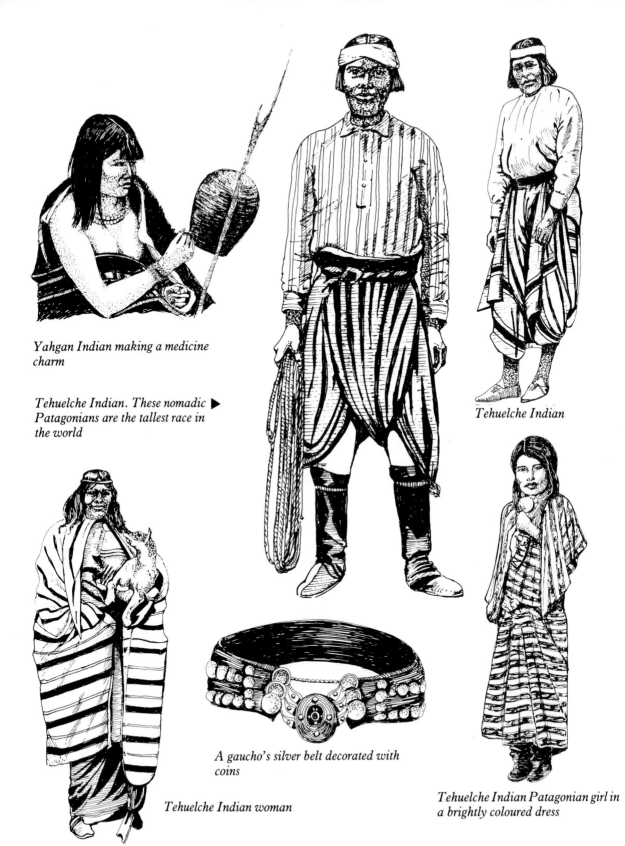

Yahgan Indian making a medicine charm

Tehuelche Indian. These nomadic ▶
Patagonians are the tallest race in the world

Tehuelche Indian

Tehuelche Indian woman

A gaucho's silver belt decorated with coins

Tehuelche Indian Patagonian girl in a brightly coloured dress

BOLIVIA

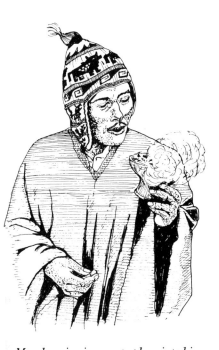

Bolivian Indian woman in a typical felt hat, possibly a copy of those worn by the early British railwaymen

Man burning incense to place into his house. He is wearing a popular knitted or woven tight-fitting helmet known as a llucho *or* chullo. *These can be plain or patterned with, for instance, stylised llamas*

Simon Bolivar, one of the 'Liberators' of South America from the Spanish, described Bolivia as 'a little marvel'. Yet there is nothing little about Bolivia. The present size is greater than France, Spain, and Portugal combined and, at the same time of Independence from Spain, it was twice that size, before all the neighbours – Argentina, Chile, Peru, Paraguay, and Brazil – took pieces from it in territorial disputes. Even so, Bolivia is the fifth largest country in South America after Brazil, Argentina, Peru, and Colombia.

Bolivia has been described as 'a microcosm of the universe' since within it are to be found every extreme of geography and climate. There are snow-capped peaks, rich fertile valleys, dense forests and tropical plains, often just a short journey apart. The climate varies from the biting cold of the Andes mountains in the west, through the temperate valleys in the centre of the country, to the humid jungles and tropical plains in the north and east.

The Andes mountains which run down the entire length of the country give Bolivia her extremes of climate and divide the country into the different regions: the highlands; the high plateau or *altiplano*; the valleys to the east of the Andes, the Yungas; the fertile semi-tropical mountain valleys; and the eastern lowlands, or *Oriente*. Seventy per cent of Bolivia's population lives in the Altiplano region. La Paz, the de facto capital city, is located there, notorious for its *sorojche*, mountain sickness, caused by the altitude and consequent lack of oxygen. The 6 million population of Bolivia is predominantly Indian. Society is clearly divided into Indians, Whites, and Cholos, a mixture of the other two races. There are three Indian groups; the Quechuas, the Aymarás, and the Guaranis. Spanish is the 'official' language but all three Indian groups maintain their own language as an integral part of their distinct culture. The Quechuas live predominantly in the Altiplano and the valleys, the Aymarás on the northern Altiplano and the Yungas. The

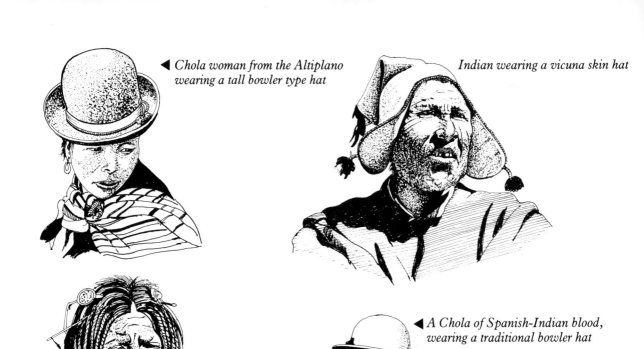

◄ *Chola woman from the Altiplano wearing a tall bowler type hat*

Indian wearing a vicuna skin hat

◄ *A Chola of Spanish-Indian blood, wearing a traditional bowler hat*

Aged Quechua woman with ornaments stuck into her plaited hair. Her warm clothes are made from the fleece of llama or vicuna

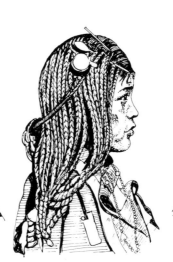

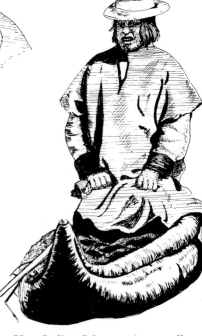

Typical Indian headdress from Carabucu in the Altiplano

Young Quechua girl with plaited hair into which ornaments and silver spoons are stuck

Urus Indian fisherman in a small reed balsa boat. These boats do not last very long as they become waterlogged

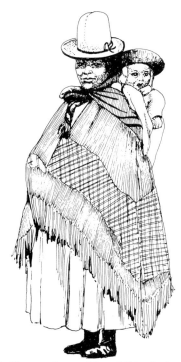

Indian mother and her child who is carried on her back in a blanket or awayo *knotted in front and worn over the shawl which is in a brightly checked colouring. It is also fringed. A derby type hat is also worn*

Guaranis make up a small population living close to the border with Paraguay. The Urus, an Indian group which lived in Bolivia at the time of Spanish colonisation, have virtually disappeared.

One of the most difficult problems for Bolivia has been that the bulk of the population is located in the poor areas of the Altiplano and not in the rich area of Oriente. Poor communication and transportation have also hindered Bolivia's development as well as maintaining the isolated position of the Indian people in Bolivian society. Bolivia has vast agricultural and mineral wealth which are only slowly being exploited.

Of the Bolivian Indians, both men and women are expert weavers, the women using the traditional hand looms, whilst the men work on a larger Spanish-type loom brought over from Europe.

The capital, La Paz, gets very cold when the sun sets, but the Cholos, well used to this, wear a warm poncho over their cotton shirts and loose trousers, and they also wear a wide-brimmed felt hat.

The women's dress is distinctly Spanish in style. Under the short skirt several brightly coloured petticoats are worn, making the skirt stand out. A shawl is worn over the shoulders, and coloured openwork stockings. There is enormous diversity in the style and colour of their hats and those, rather like tall bowlers, narrow-brimmed and made of felt, are said to be based on those worn by the early British railwaymen. The peoples living in the forest region on the banks of the Rio Grande wear white tunics made from pieces of bark, tanned and sewn together.

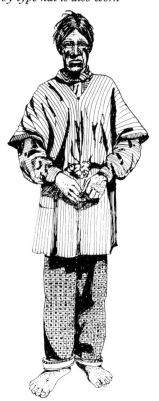

◄ *Quecha Indian in the Chipaya region. His race predominated the Inca Empire and is seen here with tribal markings on his face. He is wearing a serape or poncho with an opening at the front, and is bare-footed*

Bare-footed Indian in dark trousers and a bright sleeveless waistcoat. The hat is of felt or straw. He is playing his flute and has a small leather bag on his back

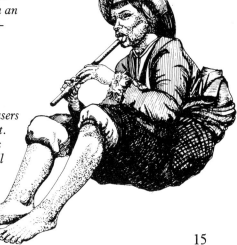

15

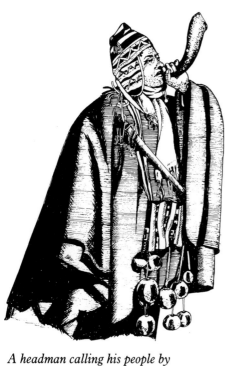

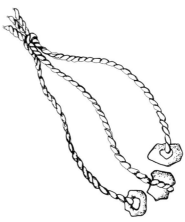

A headman calling his people by blowing on a pututu. *The woollen cap is patterned in a geometrical design and has long earflaps*

An ancient Bolivian game called liwi-liwi is played by the Aymará people. A liwi was originally used to catch creatures such as guanacos and ostriches. The game is played mainly by children throwing their liwis into the air and others trying to entangle theirs with the first

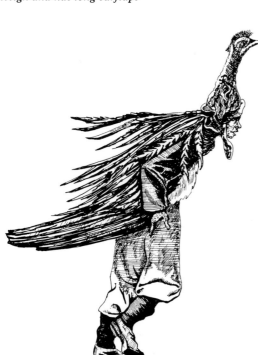

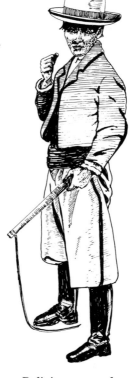

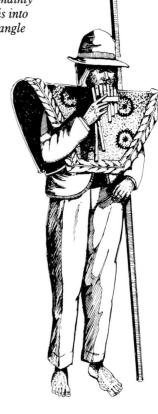

Festive costume of a birdman

Young Bolivian country boy

Festival costume worn on a feast day that ends in a general saturnalia. This man is playing a pan pipe

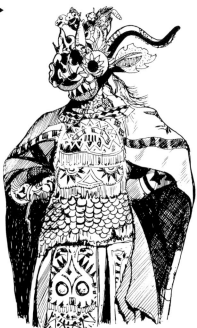

The Devil's Dance, also known as ▶ the Diablada performed at Oruro and La Paz on the Altiplano. The masks are made of plaster and painted mainly in red. They look very ferocious with twisted horns, ears with serrated edges, and bulging eyes. Jagged pieces of mirror are used for the teeth and curved to look like fangs. The foreheads are decorated with green snakes and other creatures. The belt is made of ancient coins

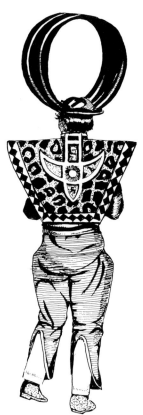

Musician's festive costume in gaudy colours with a curious slit at the back of the trousers revealing long white underpants. He is also wearing a strange circular headdress reminiscent of a drum body

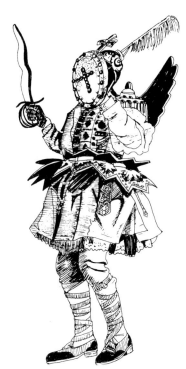

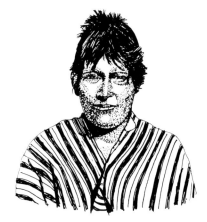

Strong Bolivian Indian of the high plateau

'Michael The Archangel' with his flaming sword. The costume like a silver-winged butterfly, is of pale blue gauze, is playing out the Diablada

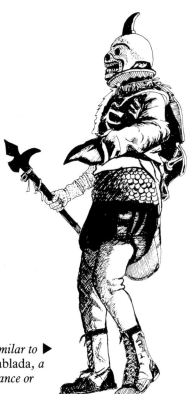

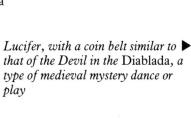

Lucifer, with a coin belt similar to ▶ that of the Devil in the Diablada, a type of medieval mystery dance or play

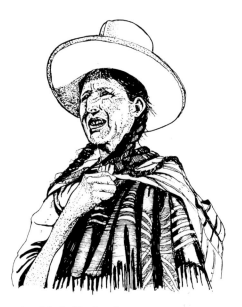

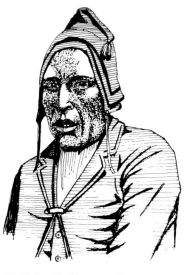

Bolivian Indian wearing a
traditional bonnet

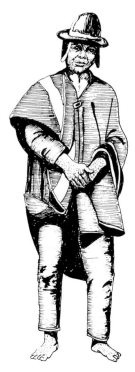

An elderly Cochamba woman
wearing a straw hat

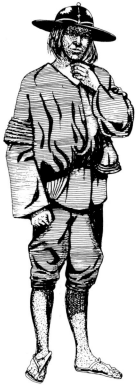

Indian man wearing a poncho and
tight-fitting woollen helmet with long
earflaps and a felt hat worn over it.
He is barefooted which is quite usual

◄ Chipaya woman wearing a style of
bowler hat, and poncho

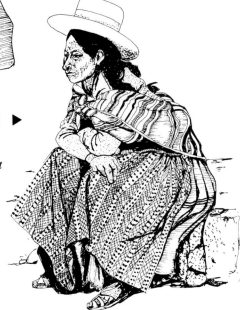

Quechua woman in a gaily patterned
skirt, under which numerous
coloured petticoats are worn. The
long sleeved blouse is also of a bright
colour, likewise the woollen shawl.
She is wearing hand-made open
leather sandals ►

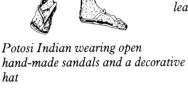

Potosi Indian wearing open
hand-made sandals and a decorative
hat

18

BRAZIL

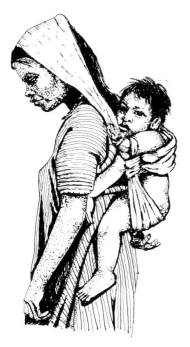

Young girl carrying water on her head. Pau de Arara are the poverty stricken peasants of the north-east

Young Brazilian Indian mother carries her baby in a sling from her head

Brazil is a continent within a continent in South America. A giant country of over 3 million square miles, almost as large an area as the United States, makes Brazil the largest tropical country in the world as well as accounting for about half the entire area of South America. The geography and climate, not surprisingly, vary enormously from the dry north-east, hit by regular droughts, to the rich forests and plains of the centre and south. Brazil is, too, a country rich in minerals with a vast agricultural potential neither of which has been realised. Such possibilities for development, economic growth and prosperity have resulted in the Brazilian expression that 'God is Brazilian'. In 1982 the population of Brazil totalled 125 million, yet two thirds of the country were virtually unoccupied. Most of Brazil's population is concentrated along the coastal area that was originally settled by Portugese colonisers, and inland in the states of Minas Gerais and São Paulo. Most of the interior of the country is sparsely populated and has yet to be developed. The founding of the new federal capital in Brazilia, deep in the interior, was a gesture from the government of the potential that existed. The lack of development has allowed the persistence of ancient cultures in the remote areas of Brazil. Whenever their pattern of living and customs have been interfered with as a result of economic developments their ancient traditions and cultures have soon been lost. The language is Portuguese and the state religion Roman Catholic.

Brazils economic history has consisted of booms followed by slumps. The sugar boom of the sixteenth and seventeenth centuries led to the import of large numbers of African slaves since the indigenous Indians were unwilling to be conscripted as labourers, forced or otherwise. By the eighteenth century sugar was in decline with coffee poised to take its place. The new crop was one of the powerful incentives to the abolition of slavery in Brazil which, in its turn, saw the rise of new interest groups in society. Rubber, in the Amazon valley, produced

19

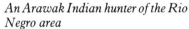
An Arawak Indian hunter of the Rio Negro area

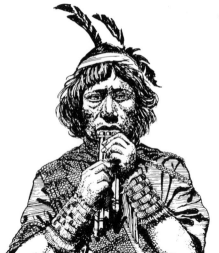

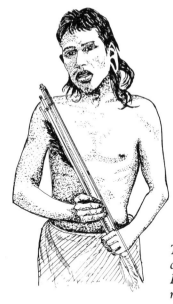

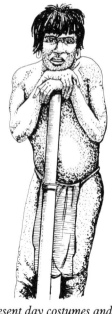

Bedecked in feathers and beads this Indian plays his reed instrument. His black hair is adorned with coloured cottons and toucan feathers. He wears fibre bracelets

The present day costumes and customs of the Arawaks, primitive Indian hunters of the Rio Negro region, differ only slightly from ancient times. Their earlobes are weighted when they are children, so by adolescence they often hang down over the shoulders

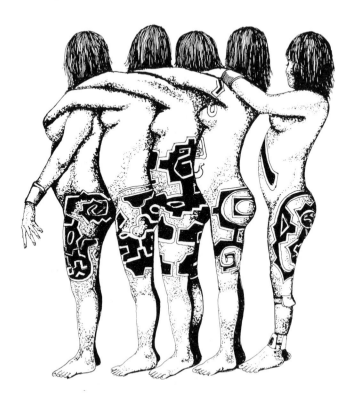

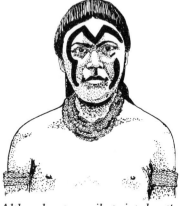

Although not so gaily painted as the women, this man of the Wauwai tribe adorned his body with coloured string and bead necklaces, painting his face with tribal markings

◄ *Amazonian girls painted in crude colours form a human snake for the strenuous dance they perform*

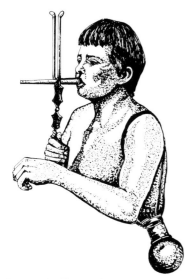

Tucuna Indian with an unusual kind of cigar holder. These tribal cigars were often used by witch doctors in their magical healing

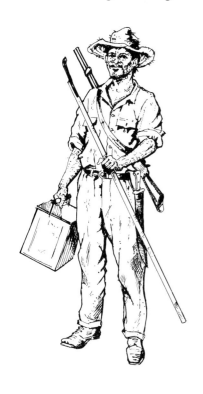

An Amazonian equipped for hunting and fishing

another short-lived boom in the late nineteenth century before it was destroyed through foreign competition. In every case Brazil's example has led to the rise of a foreign competitor resulting in slump and an unstable pattern of development. Modern Brazil's industrial developments are no exception. Brazil's booms and slumps have consistently resulted in massive immigration, both into and within the country, adding to its varied ethnic composition and bringing new influences and ideas into the country. Brazil, long regarded as the 'Sleeping Giant' of South America, and capable of Great Power status in the world, has consistently been unable to break out of its instability and take its place in the centre of the world stage.

New as the New World was to its discoverers, many expressions and names of places adopted by the Portuguese were already used by the indigenous Tupi and Guarani Indians. These people, naked and red-skinned, painted, with natural dyes, chequered designs and patterns on their faces and bodies. Indian presence is now very small. Pure-bred Indians constitute less than 1% of the population, although their facial characteristics occur in the many half-castes.

In the remoter regions the population is mainly of Indian origin, living under very primitive conditions with their own simple language. In less remote areas are to be found early Negro settlements. Brazil's four hundred years of history is in fact the story of the progressive annihilation of its original inhabitants. The remaining few have steadfastly retreated into the Amazon jungle and now live in large reservations, away from other scattered tribes that inhabit the jungle. Although some Indians have adopted Western dress, most are loathe to part with their brightly coloured beads and charms.

The Indian women of the Amazon basin bind their legs above and below the calf to create unnatural swellings and if this does not produce the desired effect, false calves of coloured clay are worn. In certain tribes the men also follow this fashion. The men shave their hair to the front and wear feathers on their heads; the feathers being obtained from the many brilliantly plumed birds which inhabit the forests.

In the depths of the forests the tribes still use a blow-pipe for killing animals. They wear little or no clothing, tattooing and painting their bodies instead. They live all their lives in a very small radius as the forests are so dense that it is only possible to travel alongside the streams. There are still traces of what seems to have been an ancient civilisation before the Spanish invasion, although the legend of the women warriors, known as

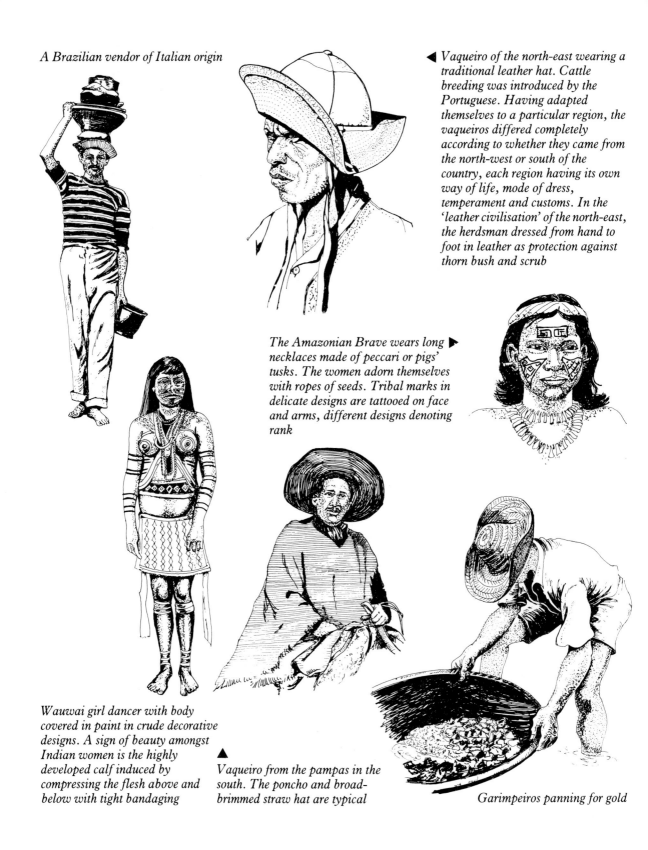

A Brazilian vendor of Italian origin

Vaqueiro of the north-east wearing a traditional leather hat. Cattle breeding was introduced by the Portuguese. Having adapted themselves to a particular region, the vaqueiros differed completely according to whether they came from the north-west or south of the country, each region having its own way of life, mode of dress, temperament and customs. In the 'leather civilisation' of the north-east, the herdsman dressed from hand to foot in leather as protection against thorn bush and scrub

The Amazonian Brave wears long ▶ necklaces made of peccari or pigs' tusks. The women adorn themselves with ropes of seeds. Tribal marks in delicate designs are tattooed on face and arms, different designs denoting rank

Wauwai girl dancer with body covered in paint in crude decorative designs. A sign of beauty amongst Indian women is the highly developed calf induced by compressing the flesh above and below with tight bandaging

Vaqueiro from the pampas in the south. The poncho and broad-brimmed straw hat are typical

Garimpeiros panning for gold

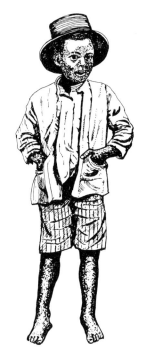

Mulatto child, a mixture of Negro and Portuguese

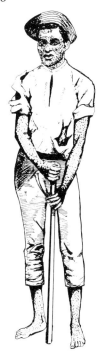

Brazilian Negro from the Minas Gerais area

Amazons, seems to be a myth. Nevertheless both boys and girls have to undergo painful initiations with uncomplaining courage before being regarded as fit members of their tribe. Only then are they permitted to take part in ceremonial dances, still popular amongst the Amazon Indians.

In preparation for the dances, also religious in concept, the Indians have to be well fed in order to be able to sustain their vigour, as these dances may continue for several days and nights. Wedding dances, for example, last non-stop for four to five days and nights, and there are always fresh performers to take place of those too exhausted to carry on. On very special occasions dances have been known to last for two weeks.

Religious processions and public ceremonies were extremely popular until the middle of the nineteenth century. The Christian festivities that preceded Lent were violent and crude, and it was not until about 1850 that carnival societies were formed and the first parades and groups took place. The change in character of the carnival with its masked balls and firework displays soon spread, becoming known as the Carnival of Rio, and giving great scope for dressing up. The Africans who came from the Congo, Nigeria and Angola, clung to their traditions from which emanated the Brazilian music, dancing and poetry. In Bahia the atabeque drums, which hail from Africa, summon people to religious ceremonies. The Bahiana women, apart from their traditional dress which includes a large turban, a full sleeved blouse and many gaily coloured skirts worn on top of each other, wear many necklaces of seeds and glass beads of many colours.

In the South are the vaqueiros, the cowboys of the pampas, who are dextrous horsemen and handle a lasso and bolas with great skill.

The dress of the vaqueiros is also characteristic, whether a foreman or a cowhand, consisting of a felt or leather hat tied beneath the chin, and a brightly coloured shirt with silk neckerchief at the throat. A broad studded belt accentuates the waist and supended from it are a revolver and a knife. The wide *bombachas*, baggy trousers, are made for easy movement. White socks turn down over the high leather boots that are adorned with large silver spurs. A poncho protects the wearer against the cold, but may also be used as a fan in fine weather. It is usually black or dark blue, made of fine wool, and flung dramatically over one shoulder to reveal the scarlet lining.

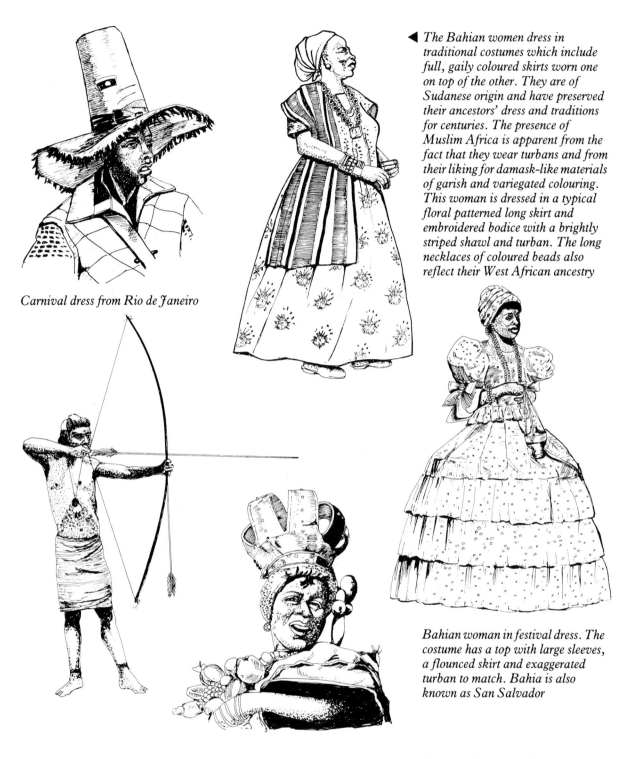

Carnival dress from Rio de Janeiro

The Bahian women dress in traditional costumes which include full, gaily coloured skirts worn one on top of the other. They are of Sudanese origin and have preserved their ancestors' dress and traditions for centuries. The presence of Muslim Africa is apparent from the fact that they wear turbans and from their liking for damask-like materials of garish and variegated colouring. This woman is dressed in a typical floral patterned long skirt and embroidered bodice with a brightly striped shawl and turban. The long necklaces of coloured beads also reflect their West African ancestry

Bahian woman in festival dress. The costume has a top with large sleeves, a flounced skirt and exaggerated turban to match. Bahia is also known as San Salvador

Bororo tribesman of the Mato Grosso taking aim with his palmwood bow

Carnival headwear. Carnivals are very popular in Brazil

CHILE

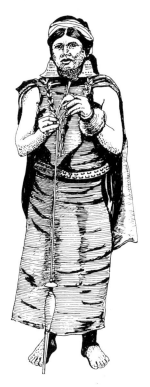

Young girl with silver ornamentation and coins in her hair. The bow would be brightly coloured

Araucanian Indian women of southern Chile. She wears few ornaments other than large earrings which are made locally of silver

Chile lies like a narrow ribbon of land between the mountains of the Andes and the Pacific Ocean. Smaller than all the other South American countries other than Ecuador, Paraguay, and Uruguay, Chile is, nevertheless, larger in area than France. Within its 4,200 km length, and average 180 km width, Chile possesses extremes of geography and climate being close to the sea and close to the Andes.

In the north in a region close to the border with Peru the geography consists of a desert of hills and plains in which Chile's nitrate and copper deposits are located. Below that there exists a semi-desert in which agriculture is carried out in valleys with the help of irrigation. In the centre of the country, where the majority of the 12 million population lives, the climate allows farms and vineyards to flourish in picturesque surroundings. Moving further south the next region has a heavy rainfall for most of the year in which dense untouched forests, and mountains alternate with agricultural land. This area is forest Chile. The southern-most region is made up of mountains, forests, islands, and channels. Few people live in this inhospitable, icy, stormy, climate.

For three centuries of Spanish occupation of Chile there existed continual wars between the Mapuche Indians, the indigenous population, and the Spanish colonisers. Not until the nineteenth century could immigrants settle in the Mapuche lands in the south. Today, most Chilean Indians, some 150 thousand of them, live in the forest lands around Temuco between the Bio-Bio and the Toltén rivers. Most of the population is now *mestizo*, of mixed European and Indian blood. Just 5% of the population is European. In the nineteenth century immigrants from Germany, Italy, France, Switzerland, Britain and East Europe all made their mark on the culture of the country. Their influence on Chile is far out of proportion to their numbers. Most Chileans, live in towns and cities reflecting the trend towards a move from the land to the towns.

25

Chile changed most dramatically in the nineteenth century as it became increasingly caught up in trade with the rest of the world. First, the Californian gold rush gave a temporary boom to agriculture. But it was Chile's mineral assets which provided the most sustained wealth. By 1870 Chile controlled a quarter of the world market in copper which, although to decline, rose again in the twentieth century to remain Chile's most important single export. Nitrates, for explosives and fertilisers, were the leading exports until after the First World War when they declined against competition with synthetic chemicals. The growth of these industries, and sometimes their decline, led to important social and cultural changes in Chile; new centres of power, growing urbanisation, the introduction of new ideas and values, and the growth of new classes.

Roman Catholicism was the state religion until 1925 when the church was disestablished.

Women's traditional costumes are full skirted over which they wear long sleeved jackets or blouses. A shawl or blanket usually of red or dark blue, is worn around the shoulders and knotted in front. They have black, shiny, coarse hair which they wear in two long plaits down their backs, with the simple adornment of a high comb.

The huasos ride on high pommelled saddles ornamented with silver, wearing brightly coloured red and yellow ponchos, many handwoven from the silky hair of llama or guanaco. The

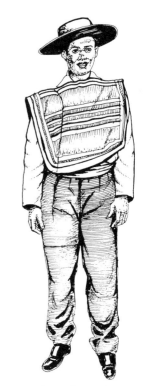

Huaso wearing a broad-brimmed hat made of felt. A short colourful poncho covers the shoulders, back and chest. It is worn over a jacket

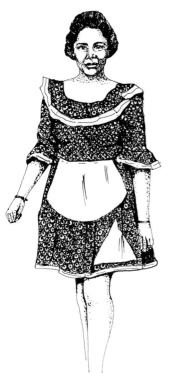

◀ *Chilean girl dressed in a traditional festive costume performing the cueca, a national dance*

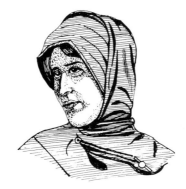

Woman wearing the traditional manto *drawn over her head and fastened at the neck*

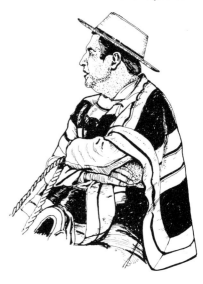

Huaso wearing a brightly coloured large poncho

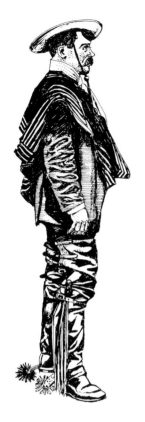

dress of the indigenous Chileans, the Mapuches, has become more European of recent years, especially that of the men who prefer more sombre colours than the women. Traditionally, however, they wore a *chamanto* or blanket caught between the legs like trousers and fastened to a belt, falling like a skirt. Some still wear this type of garment today, called a *chirpà*, which is crossed between the legs and fastened to the belt, or they may wear very wide trousers, *charahuilla*, tied at the ankles.

Women also wear the chamanto fastened at the shoulders, covering the body down to the ankles with a woollen sash around the waist. A cloak of the same material can also be worn, falling from the shoulders and held at the neckline by a silver clasp.

Before the Spanish Conquest stones and shells formed the basis of their finery, glass beads taking their place later on, and, comparatively recently, silver came into use. They wear necklaces and rings, bracelets and anklets, and woollen bands with silver ends may be worn in their plaited hair. In the Chilean archipelego it was the women who gathered shellfish on the beaches at low tide or who, from bark canoes, dived into the water with a shell blade and a basket held in their teeth. They carried a fire on a clay platform in their canoes, both for warmth and for roasting the shellfish over the coals. The men hunted cormorants and other sea birds and harpooned seals and whales.

This huaso's trousers are tucked into long black gaiters or leggings which are worn over black boots or shoes. They are fastened with buckles at the sides and round the knees are bands from which hang long leather tassels. His hat is held on with a chin band. Under the poncho or chamanto, which is folded back, a jacket is worn

The manto, *a typical Chilean ▶ feature of women's costume and a development of the Spanish mantilla, consists of a long narrow piece of black material draped over the head, around the face, and folded and pinned at the neckline, the remainder hanging down to the feet*

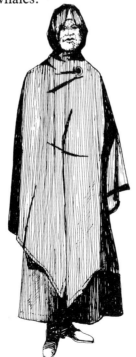

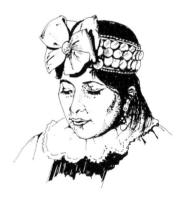

Headdress of silver design with silver coins tied with a bow in front. These headdresses are worn on festive occasions

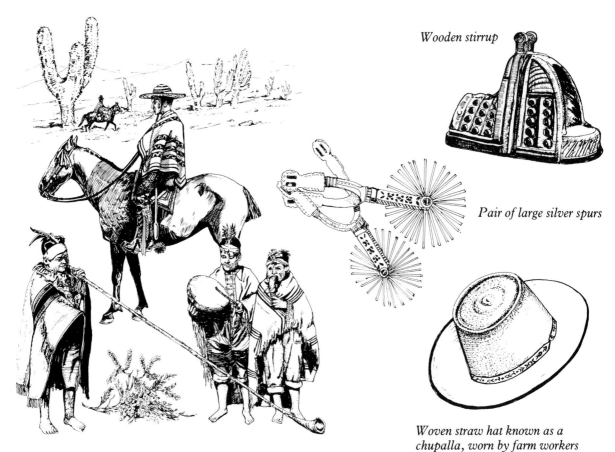

Wooden stirrup

Pair of large silver spurs

Woven straw hat known as a chupalla, worn by farm workers

The landscape is typical of Chile where the hills are covered with cacti. The estanciero, or landowner, is seen in his traditional decorative costume. The poncho or chamanto is shorter than that of the Argentinians, but the silver spurs are larger. In the foreground are Mapuche children in traditional costume playing music around a sacred branch

Typical example of Quinchamali pottery with lamp black applied to the clay

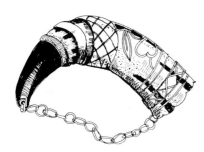

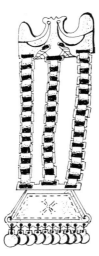

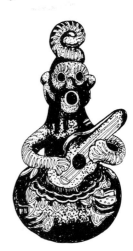

Breast ornament hung with silver coins, known as a tapu. This is a distinctive feature of the Araucanian women and is usually three stranded based on old Inca designs

Cow horn

COLOMBIA

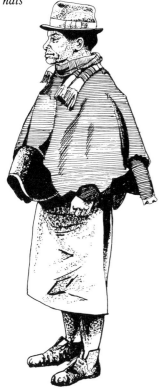

Guambiano woman hand spinning wool. In common with all Andean people, both men and women wear felt hats

Guambiano man with a type of poncho called a ruana. *Over the knee-length trousers a skirt, slightly longer, is worn*

Colombia, in the extreme north west of South America, is the fourth largest country in the continent. Despite having a foot in both the Pacific and Atlantic Oceans Colombia is an isolated country made more so by her geographical and climate differences. Each part of Colombia has its own distinct and particular character. More than half of the country is virtually uninhabited, the rest living in the most mountainous part of the country. Colombia's nearly 28 million population is spread throughout the country; some areas, like Antioquia and Caldas, are predominantly European; Pasto is Indian, with the Canea Valley and the area on the Caribbean coast African or *mulatto*, European and African. Colour prejudice and discrimination are strong in parts of Colombia.

Indian groups occupied Colombia long before the arrival of the Spanish. In the eastern Cordillera of the Andes dense tribes of Chibcha Indians, totalling a million people, lived settled agricultural lives producing mostly maize and potatoes. Their chief god, like the Incas, was the sun which they represented in gold artifacts. Numerous other Indian groups (the Tairona, Quimbaya, Sinú, and Calima) had established their cultures in pre-Columbian Colombia.

Colombia is the land of the mythical El Dorado. The legend claims that whenever a new Chibcha chief came to power, this marked by an elaborate ceremony of anointing him and covering him entirely in gold dust, and plunging him into the sacred lake Guatavita, one of many sacred places, and then tossing gold and precious stones in the lake after him. The name El Dorado means The Golden One.

The Chibcha who lived in the central highlands were more highly developed than most other tribes. They were mostly miners, farmers and craftsmen and left many hand-wrought artifacts, mainly of gold and other precious metals.

Apart from the warlike Caribs, who inhabited the Atlantic coast and shores of the Magdalena River, Colombian Indian tribes are very similar to each other. Spanish is the official

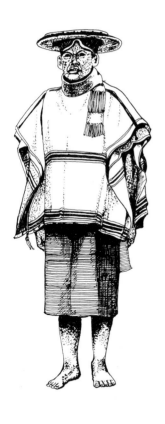

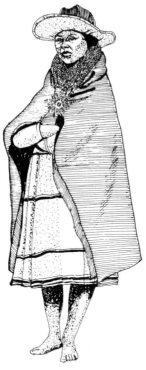

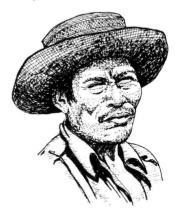

◀◀ *Guambiano man in wedding costume, barefooted*

◀ *Guambiano woman in wedding costume. Her shawl is the same bright blue as most men's shirts. The number of glass beaded necklaces worn, bought from the Putumayo area, denote wealth*

Man of the Cubeo tribe

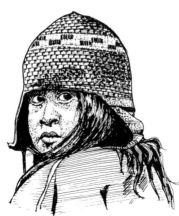

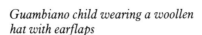

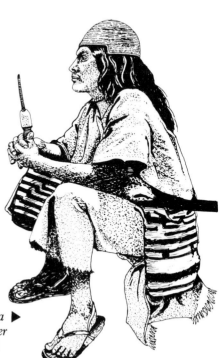

Guambiano child wearing a woollen hat with earflaps

Guambiano child

Archuaca man with a woollen cap, a poncho and striped mochila on either side. Another one is usually carried at the back as well ▶

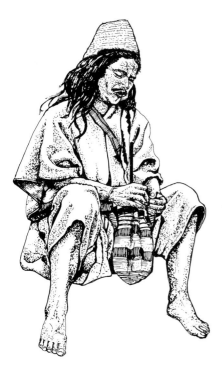

Archuaca man wearing a woollen hat, wide trousers and a poncho. He has a mochola or bag, in front of him. He is barefooted

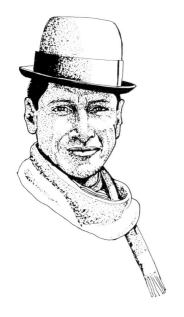

Guambiano man with a felt hat shaped like a trilby

language spoken by all but a few Indians who live in remoter regions. The population is mainly made up of Mestizos of mixed and European blood, pure European ancestry, Mulatto, Negro and a few Zambo-mixed Negro and Indian. The pure Indians are fast disappearing. The Negros originally imported from Africa as slaves by the Spaniards now live mainly in the hotter regions.

The Archuaca live on the western slopes of the Sierra Nevada. The women spend a great deal of their time knitting, spinning and making clothes. They also weave *mochilas*, the traditional native carrying bags. These have a special significance for them as they receive an unfinished one on their marriage. Also during visits to each other, women often exchange with each other the ones that they are in the midst of weaving for either their husbands or fiancés. The mochila is usually in brown and white stripes and an important part of dress. Three of these bags are normally carried, one on each side crossed over each other and a third which hangs from the neck down the back and holds coca (leaves for chewing).

The Archuaca usually wear hats of wool or cotton which are generally in white with fertility symbols, such as green frogs, sewn on. The men wear wide trousers that reach below the knees and a poncho which is tied around the waist with a white woollen or cotton belt decorated with black or coloured stripes to match those down the centre of the poncho, and trousers. Women wear two white knee-length tunics or robes. One of the tunics is slit up the left side and the other on the right, giving the appearance of a dress without any opening. They also wear woollen or cotton belts, and *chaquira* necklaces which are elegantly interwoven, as well as a *mochila* which hangs from the forehead down the back.

Young girls wear simple knee-length dresses tied with a small cloth belt, and small boys a tunic, generally made from two of their mother's old robes, with a V-shaped collar.

The Cubeos who live mainly in the west of Colombia, wear multi-coloured feathers on their bodies and as a headdress for their ceremonies. This tribe is more masculine orientated, women being excluded from certain rites and ceremonies.

On the western slopes of the central mountain range live the Guambianos who have preserved their own language. The men wear white knee-length trousers, and over them a bright blue skirt which is also knee length and held up by a leather belt. They usually wear Western type shirts, brightly coloured with long sleeves, and have one or two traditional ponchos in black, white or grey, which can also be used as a covering at night.

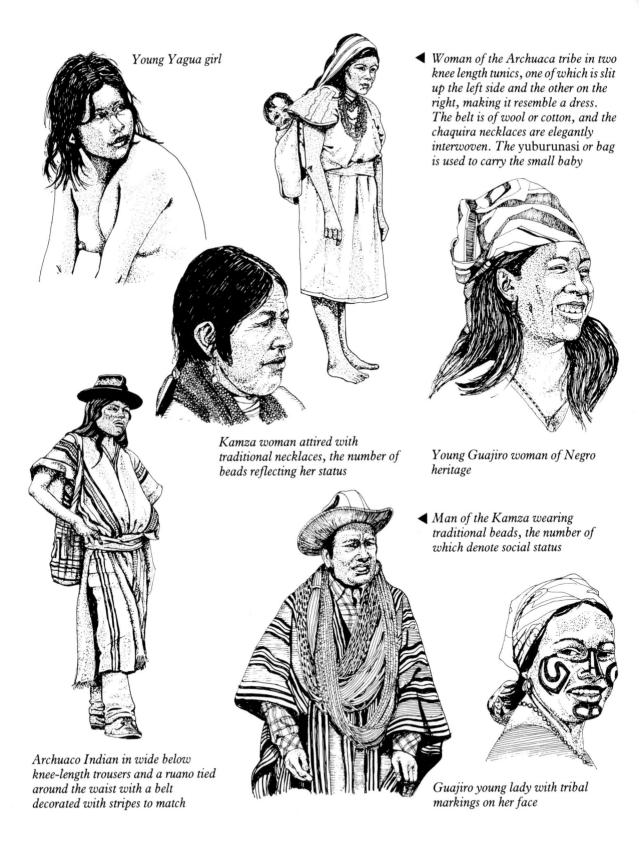

Young Yagua girl

Woman of the Archuaca tribe in two
knee length tunics, one of which is slit
up the left side and the other on the
right, making it resemble a dress.
The belt is of wool or cotton, and the
chaquira necklaces are elegantly
interwoven. The yuburunasi or bag
is used to carry the small baby

Kamza woman attired with
traditional necklaces, the number of
beads reflecting her status

Young Guajiro woman of Negro
heritage

Man of the Kamza wearing
traditional beads, the number of
which denote social status

Archuaco Indian in wide below
knee-length trousers and a ruano tied
around the waist with a belt
decorated with stripes to match

Guajiro young lady with tribal
markings on her face

PLATE 1, ARGENTINA   The Tehuelche Indian of Patagonia, bottom right, is dressed in bright colours and similarly to those of the northern area. The Ona Indian from the Tierra del Fuego, on the extreme left, is wearing a guanaco skin over one shoulder, covering the remainder of his body. The bow and arrow was the main hunting weapon. In summer he generally wears no clothing at all. The top right shows the Spanish influence in dance costume, which is very popular in Argentina. The gaucho in the centre holds a stiletto, a most essential item in his equipment, and a silver bombilla from which he drinks his maté. The wide leather belt is ornamented with silver coins and other decorations and has a heavy silver buckle. Wrapped around his waist he has a square garment or chirpá

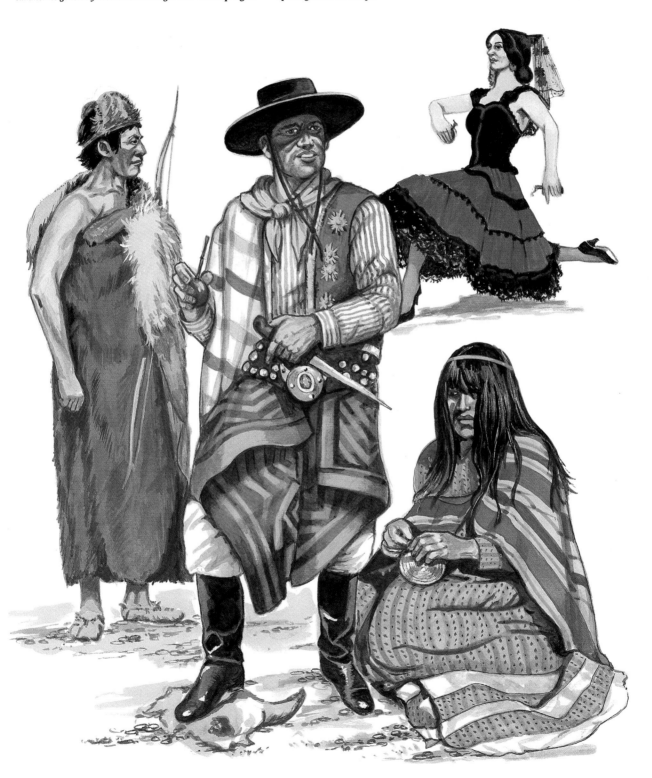

PLATE 2, BRAZIL *The vaquero or cowhand of the north-east is dressed from head to foot in leather. His leather hat is shown in the left foreground.* The woman from Bahia, front right, is dressed in a traditional costume that includes brightly coloured full skirts, one worn over the other. These Baianas are of Sudanese origin and have preserved their traditional dress for centuries. Being prominently of African origin, she wears a turban. The little girl is in a patchwork dress. Top left *is a man dressed for a dance contest, the copoera, which is a major attaction in the streets of Salvador, Bahia, during large festivals.* The gaucho, top right, *a borderer from the south, in his characteristic dress. His broad brimmed hat of either felt or leather could be tied beneath his chin, and he wears a kerchief around his neck. His broad belt has a revolver and a knife suspended from it. His socks fall over his boots which are always adorned with large spurs*

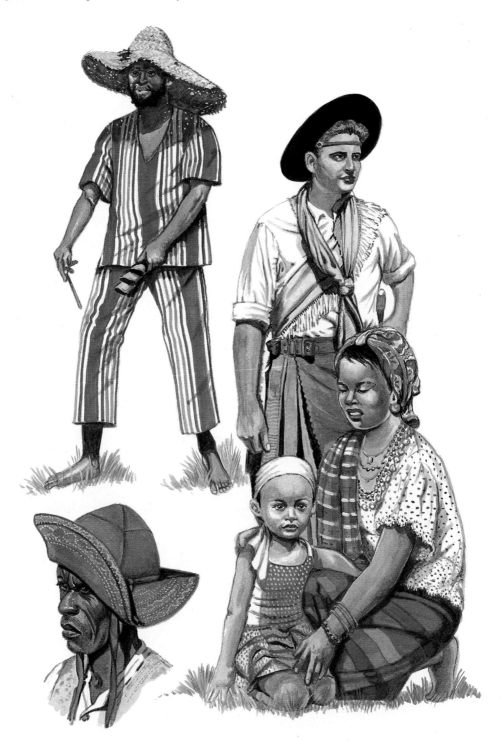

PLATE 3, CHILE   In the foreground is a Mapuche or Araucanian in traditional costume. The silver chain hung with silver coins is based on Inca designs, and is known as a tapu. The silver coin bedecked headdress is tied on with coloured bows. Black is commonly worn. The Chilean cowboy or huaso in the centre is dressed similarly to the cowboys in other South American countries with slight distinctive features. He is wearing long black trousers, a wide-brimmed hat, held in place with a leather strap, and his short poncho is in multi-coloured stripes. The girl on the right is wearing an adaptation of western style dress, whilst the shepherd in the background is in the ever-popular poncho

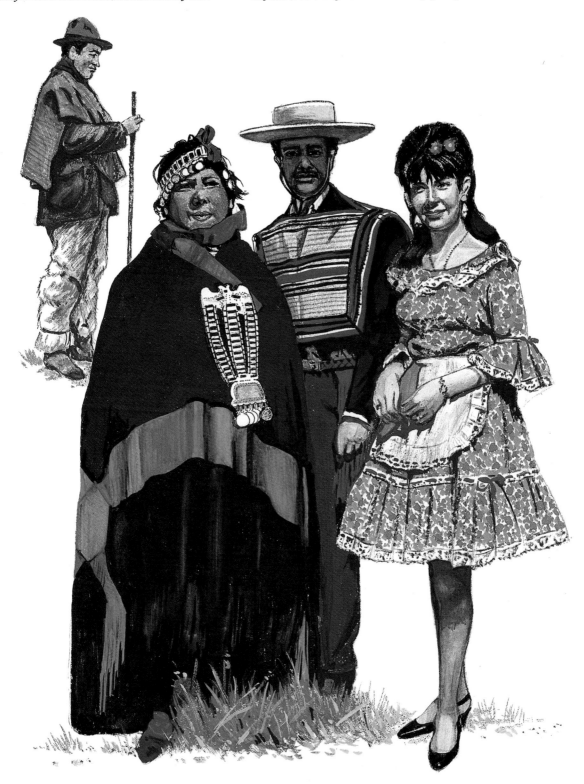

PLATE 4, COLOMBIA   On the left is a Guambiano bridegroom in his wedding outfit which consists of a double layered white and striped ruana. He is also wearing a coloured scarf around his neck. Over his close-fitting skull cap he wears a large felt circular hat. The bright blue skirt is a noteable feature amongst Guambiano men. Like most, this man is bare-footed. On the right is a shepherd from the Arhuaco tribe, wearing a close fitting cap, a tunic with short, loose wide sleeves and trousers that end just above the ankles. Over this he is wearing a poncho. He has three mochillas or bags, one either side and the third hung around the neck at the back. He is sucking on the poporo which contains lime from crushed seashells. Coca, a form of cocaine, can also be chewed. Sitting on a mule, a popular form of transport, is a young Guajiro girl wearing a long loose flowered dress. She wears a colourful headscarf, and her face is painted with tribal markings. The young man in the background is wearing a poncho in a striped design

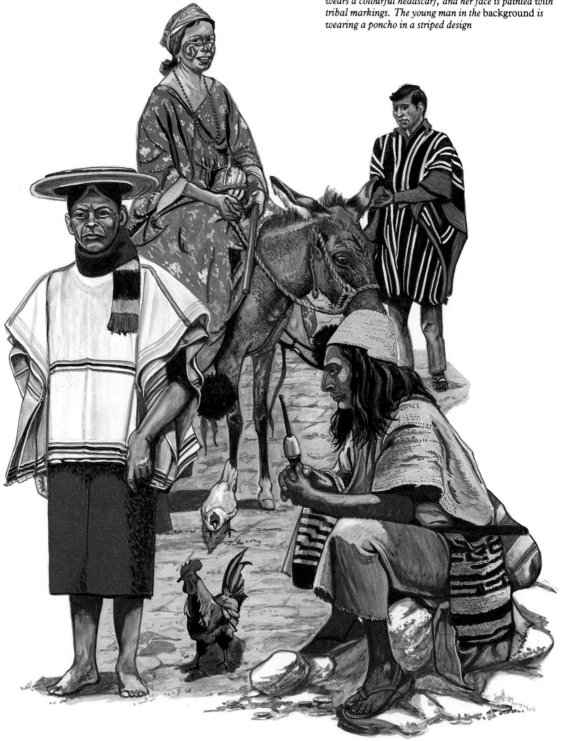

PLATE 5, ECUADOR   In the foreground sits a young Colorado Indian girl wearing a simple wrap-around skirt, and a shawl over her shoulders. Her face and body are painted in dark stripes. She is seen here picking the achiota berries to make the red dye used by the men for their hair and body decoration. At the back, on the left the Jivaro Indian warrior has his long hair decorated with a feathered headdress made of toucan feathers. Long strings of beads adorn his neck and are placed around his body. A shrunken head is also hanging around his neck. He is wearing a striped skirt and carries a spear made of the hard wood of the chonta tree. A young Corfanes Indian boy, centre back, is wearing a crown of toucan feathers. He also wears feathers stuck through his earlobes and nose. Masses of rows of beads are entwined around his neck with a necklace of animals' teeth to his shoulders. The simple shirt reaches the knees. On the right, the flute player, from the Otavalo province, is wearing a wide felt hat. Over his simple white cotton shirt and three-quarter length trousers he is wearing a poncho, popular throughout South America. The woman on the left has her small child in a shawl which is slung over her shoulders, giving her more freedom of movement

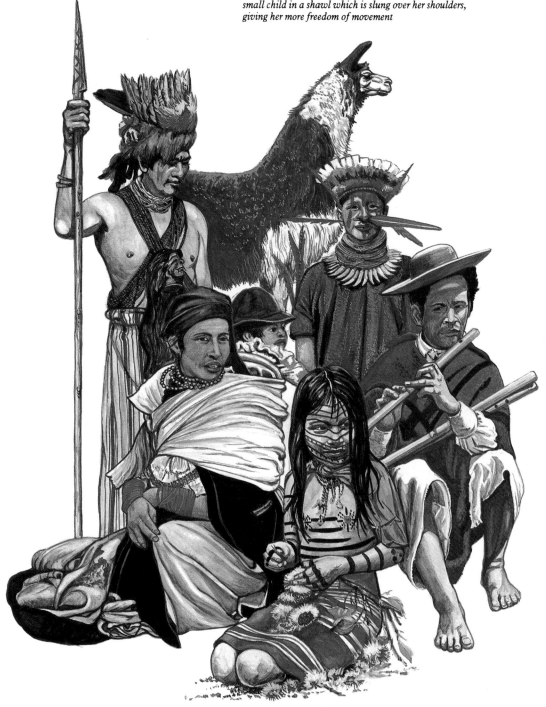

PLATE 6, BOLIVIA/PERU   The Peruvian Amahuaca Indian woman on the right, with a baby in a shawl slung over one shoulder, is covered in tribal markings. Across the top part of the face these are painted in such a way as to resemble a fine veil. Even the baby is painted. The body paint comes from two fruits, the red-orange achiota and the purple-black huito. Apart from being decorative, achiota is considered insect repellent. There are few set designs, the patterns being left to the discretion of the artist. The Peruvian Amahuaca Indian man, at the back, is wearing a tall hat made of the inner layers of bamboo covered by strips of finely woven cloth soaked in achiota and covered with black and dark red seeds interspersed with monkey teeth. A coarse fringe of shredded bast around the base of the hat can hang over the eyes. He wears a bark belt under a large stomacher made of seeds that could be as much as 45 metres in length, and a knee-length fringed skirt of red dyed cotton strings. He is also wearing a nasal disc. These were originally made from triangular pieces of tortoiseshell or mother-of-pearl, but could also be a silver coin. The Peruvian in the background is wearing a brightly coloured poncho over a shirt and dark trousers. His headwear consists of a knitted chullo and he is holding the brightly coloured flat hat in his hand. The Bolivian woman, behind the large hand-made earthenware pot, is from Tarabuco, and is bedecked in silver coins and ornaments, whilst the one in the foreground, a Chola or mestizo, is wearing the typical type of hat, sometimes made of cardboard

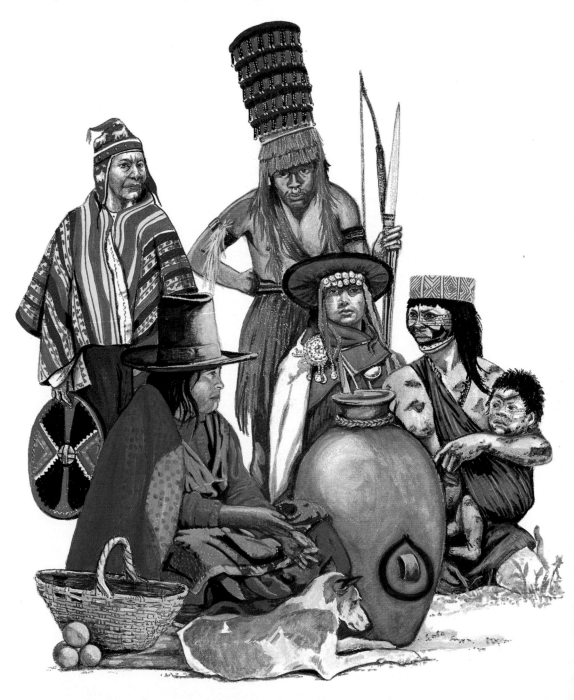

PLATE 7, PARAGUAY/URAGUAY The Paraguayan harp player is wearing a poncho. Paraguay is famous for this type of instrument and is known as the Land of the Harp. On the left the young Paraguayan girl is wearing a traditional costume for the dance known as 'La Chiperita'. The flimsy black blouse has long white patterned lace sleeves. The off-the-shoulder collar is black with white embroidery. The full, flared white skirt has a decorative motif just above the deep decorated base. She is wearing long strings of beads as well as flowers in her hair. In the centre, the young Uraguayan girl, of European-Spanish origin is wearing a natural wool poncho and a large sombrero type felt hat. The typical Uraguayan gaucho on the right is wearing a large-brimmed felt hat fastened under the chin with a leather strap. The coloured neckerchief is tucked into the open-necked checked shirt. The full woollen trousers, gathered at the ankles, are held up by a broad belt. The trousers are tucked into riding boots. The horse harness held in his hand is, as is common, decorated with silver. The chiripá, a large woollen shawl, often worn around the waist with the corners between the legs, is seen here folded and carried over his shoulder

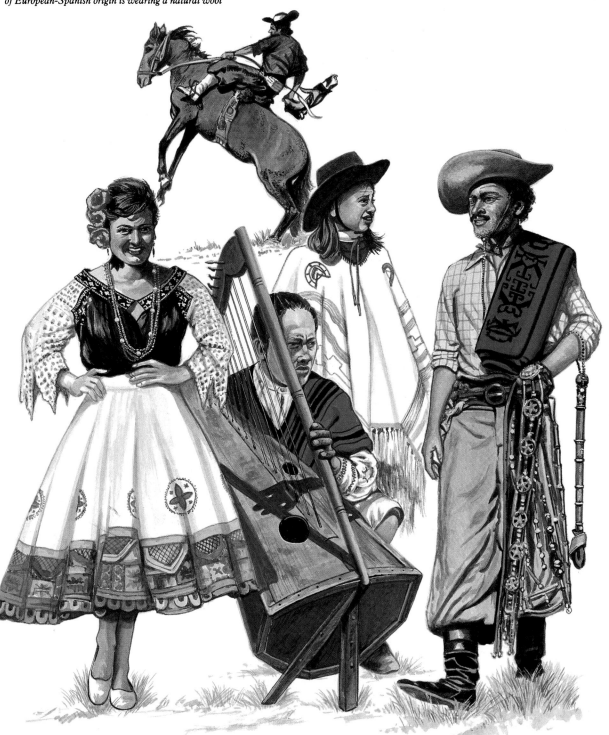

PLATE 8, VENEZUELA/GUYANA   The west
Venezuelan Indian woman in the centre is of the Guajiro
tribe, dressed in bright colours, and her face is covered with
tribal markings. The Venezuelan man in the foreground left
is wearing a horizontal striped shirt with a colourful knotted
neckerchief. The white trousers can be rolled up to the calves,
and the large straw hat has a turned-up brim. The girl, top
left, is from the Guyana plateau bordering on to Brazil. She
is painted in tribal designs on her face and body. The
Amazonian man from Guyana top right, is also painted in
his tribal designs. On the bottom right the Negro woman
from Guyana is seen wearing the familiar topi to ward off the
heat of the sun

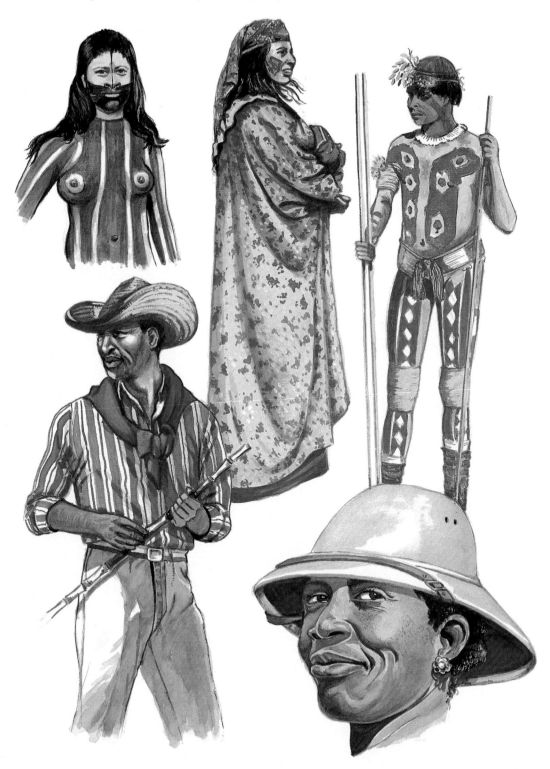

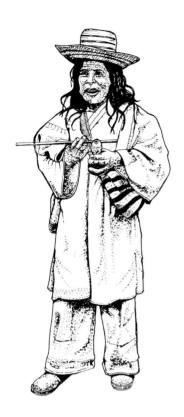

Kogui man

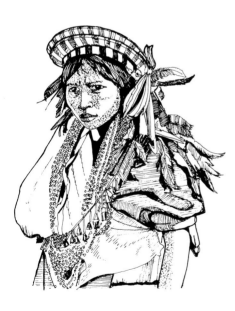

Kamza girl in a festive costume

Women wear brightly coloured short-sleeved blouses and shawls, and black pleated skirts with coloured stripes. A white cloth belt or *chumbe*, decorated with coloured paintings, is also popular. The amount and weight of their jewellery, usually of glass beads bought from the Indians of the Putumayo area, reflects the prestige of the wearer.

The men play flutes, horns and drums, whilst the women carry rattles in their hands and around their necks. The Kamza tribe who live in the valley of Sibundoy, celebrate with a carnival three days before Ash Wednesday. They perform traditional dances and songs. It is the biggest celebration of the year and a great deal of time is spent making their brilliantly coloured costumes as well as their instruments. Their traditional necklaces reflect their status by the number of beads used.

Of the Indians which inhabit the mountainous lands of the Sierra Nevada range, the men knit their own clothing with the yarn they buy from the white man, and the women make their dresses which consist of a rectangular piece of cloth folded around the body, with a belt around the waist and knotted on the left.

A small group of Yagua Indians are semi-nomadic and inhabit the Peruvian and Columbian Amazon areas. They make their own clothes from leaves of the chamba palm. The women's dress is called the *paruma*.

The native make dress covers the body from the shoulders to the upper thigh and includes a type of palm garter for their arms and legs.

The Yaguas protect their skin with various oils taken from the native plants. They are superstitious and use amulets and talismans of seed covered with fine threads from the chambira palm. They are very able musicians, the instruments mainly being percussive and vibratory. They are essentially hunters and fishermen and their main source of income is from their handcrafts.

In the Latin-American tradition, the Colombians as a whole are fond of singing and dancing. As many as 40 carnivals are held annually, with floats, masquarades, dance contests, fireworks and hurdy-gurdy players, and the shaking of maracas. Whilst the culture is mainly Spanish, many Negro and Indian customs are interwoven.

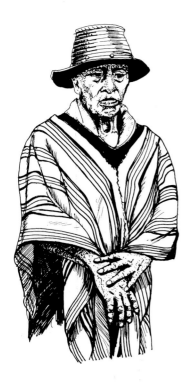

Old man of the Kamza area wearing a striped poncho

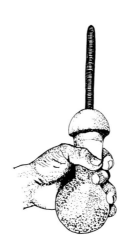

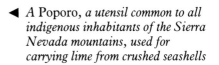

Inga man drinking chicha, a fermented corn beer

◄ A Poporo, *a utensil common to all indigenous inhabitants of the Sierra Nevada mountains, used for carrying lime from crushed seashells*

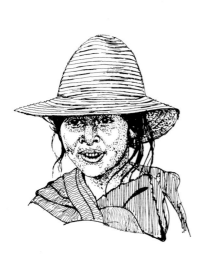

Inga woman in a straw hat

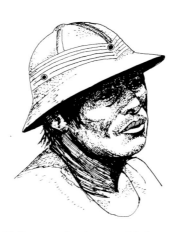

Cubean worker in a moulded sun helmet

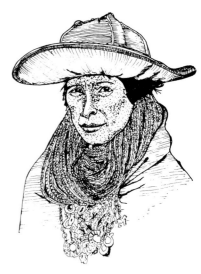

Kamza woman attired with traditional necklaces, the number of beads reflecting her status

ECUADOR

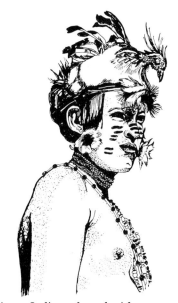

Jivaro Indian with feather headdress carrying a spear made of a hard black wood

Jivaro Indian adorned with toucan feathers and long strings of beads

Ecuador takes its name from the fact that the equator runs just a few kilometres north of Quito, the country's capital. Bordered by Colombia to the north, Peru to the east and South and the Pacific ocean to the west, Colombia is the second smallest republic in South America. The Andes mountains run from Colombia in the north to Peru in the south forming a mountainous spine through Ecuador. The mountainous area, made up of two ranges, is known as the Sierra. Here, temperature, and climate generally, depends upon altitude. Throughout the Sierra are basins in which settlement and agriculture have been possible. More than half provide pasture for sheep and cattle, in others hardy crops like potatoes are grown along with maize, wheat, barley fruit, and vegetables. Nearly half the population live in the trough between the two mountain ranges of the Andes, the Indian population live in the Andes valleys.

Many Indians live at subsistence level maintaining centuries-old styles of life and customs with little contact with the rest of society. A minority are developing traditional skills and crafts. For most Indians their lot is one of unremitting toil. The system known as *huasipungo* (from the Quechua word *puncu*, meaning door; these are the workers who sleep behind their master's door) still exists whereby the Indian works as a serf on his master's land in return for a tiny plot of his own.

The other region of Ecuador, the *Costa*, consists of the coastal areas which are an important agricultural zone. Nearly half the population live here, almost the same amount in the Sierra. Of the 8 million population 40% are Indian, 40% *mestizo*, 10% Europeans, the rest consisting of Black and Asian people.

As the climate is so warm, clothes are of little importance during the day but it gets cool at night so a poncho is necessary. In contrast to the sunny outside in the daytime the interiors of buildings is usually cool and for this reason, men have a habit of keeping their hats on indoors after the courtesy of raising them when they enter.

The poncho is part of the traditional costume, complete with wide-brimmed straw hat, the only headwear which is worn by men as well as women. Their skill in straw weaving produces some of the best and cheapest panama hats in the world made from the toquilla plant which is easily grown in the hot and damp climate. Cotton and wool from which ponchos and other warm garments are produced are spun on very simple looms by the women.

The traditional way for mothers to carry their children is in a shawl slung over their shoulders, giving the mothers freedom of movement. Dress is generally simple. Linen trousers are very popular although the Napo Indians, for example, prefer long white shirts. Generally ornamentation consists of feathers, beads and necklaces made of animal teeth, or buttons made from vegetable ivory – the insides of large nuts – which becomes hard and white. Some tribes paint their bodies whilst others make beautiful costumes from the plumage of exotic birds.

The Jivaros, the most savage of the Indian tribes, are small peoples, and inhabit the south east of the country. The men wear their hair long, ornamented with red and yellow toucan feathers. The head-hunters of this tribe wear bamboo shoots in their ears, and necklaces made of white buttons. Even today

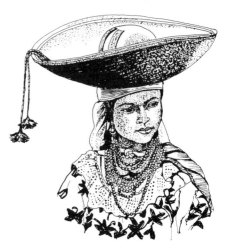

A wedding costume of the Otavala province with masses of jewellery

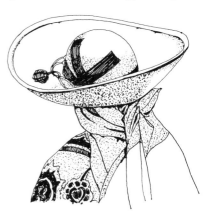

Back view of a felt hat worn at a wedding by an Otavalos Indian

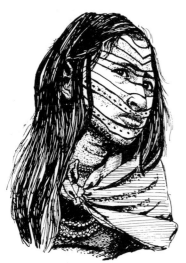

Young Colorado girl. The facial ornamentation is not tattooed but painted with natural dyes, having to be frequently renewed

Indian wearing poncho made of the ▶ *finest wool that is raised in the highlands around Quito*

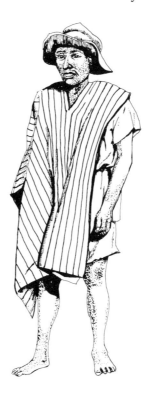

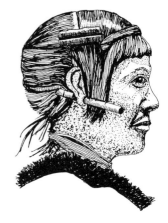

Jivaro Indian hairstyle with bamboo earrings through his lobes

36

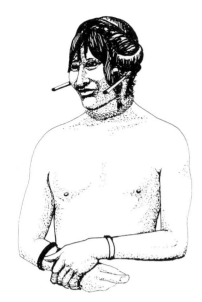

Jivaro Indian head-hunter with bamboo tubes in his ears and a necklace of white vegetable ivory buttons

they are still unwilling to disclose the mysterious method of shrinking a human head to the size of a clenched fist. All that is known is that a special drug is used. The shrunken head is known as a *tsantza*.

In the highlands in the west of Pichincha Province live the peace-loving Colorados tending their pigs. The men wear the brightest colours, their hair stained red with achota, which is the boiled down liquid of a berry, and the hair is then cut in the shape of a cap and greased to give it a brilliance.

To compensate for the brightly coloured clothes and toucan feather ornamentation of the men, the women paint extra colours on their hands and stain their teeth blue.

All this ornamentation is painted, not tattooed, so has to be renewed periodically. The Colorados have frequent festivals where they drink sugar-cane brandy to such an extent that their health is adversely affected.

There are many fiestas in Ecuador with fantastic, gaudy and garlanded effigies carried by the Indians with the processions attended by dancers and masquaraders, the men dressed in brightly coloured ponchos, and the women in multi-coloured shawls.

Jivaro Indian with his long hair ▶ *ornamented with red and yellow toucan feathers at the back*

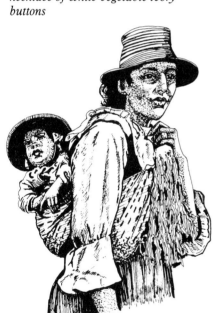

Ecuadorian woman with her small child and a shawl slung over her shoulder. In this way the mother is free to do other things

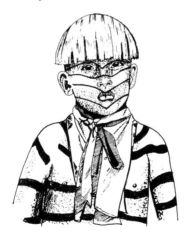

Colorado Indian with his hair stiffened and stained with achota berry juice. The hair is covered with a grease like vaseline to give it brilliance

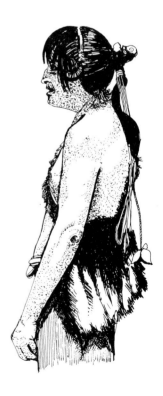

37

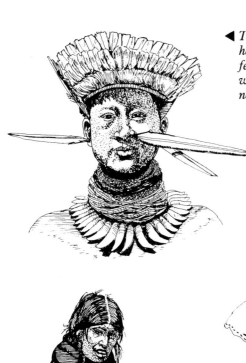

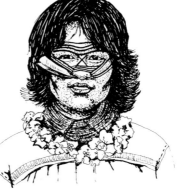

◀ *This Indian from the Cofanes group has bedecked himself with toucan feathers. Around his neck he is wearing coloured beads and a necklace made of vegetable ivory*

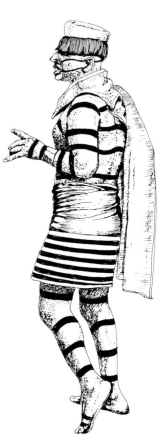

Girl from the Cofane with feathers and tribal markings

Colorados Indian dressed for a festive occasion. His hair is stained red with achota berry juice and cut in the shape of a cap. His body is painted with natural dyes

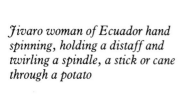

Jivaro woman of Ecuador hand spinning, holding a distaff and twirling a spindle, a stick or cane through a potato

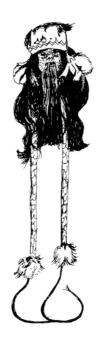

Jivaro Indians of the tropical forests ▶ have shrunken heads, this being an example, in order to obtain supernatural powers. As these powers gradually fade the heads must constantly be replenished

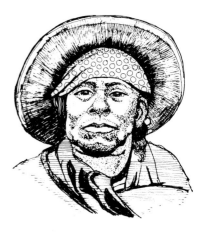

Popular hat made of panama

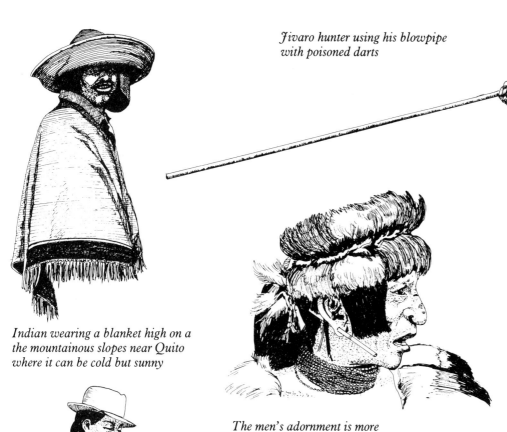

Jivaro hunter using his blowpipe with poisoned darts

Indian wearing a blanket high on the mountainous slopes near Quito where it can be cold but sunny

The men's adornment is more elaborate than that of the women. This man is bedecked in toucan feathers, a bamboo stick through his earlobe and rows of beads around his neck

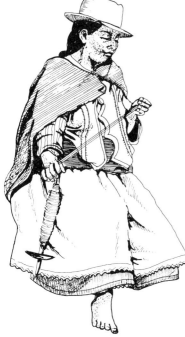

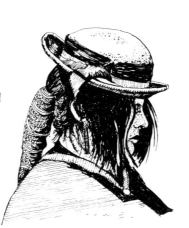

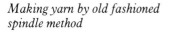

Young Jivaro girl

A straw hat made from the toquilla plant

Making yarn by old fashioned spindle method

39

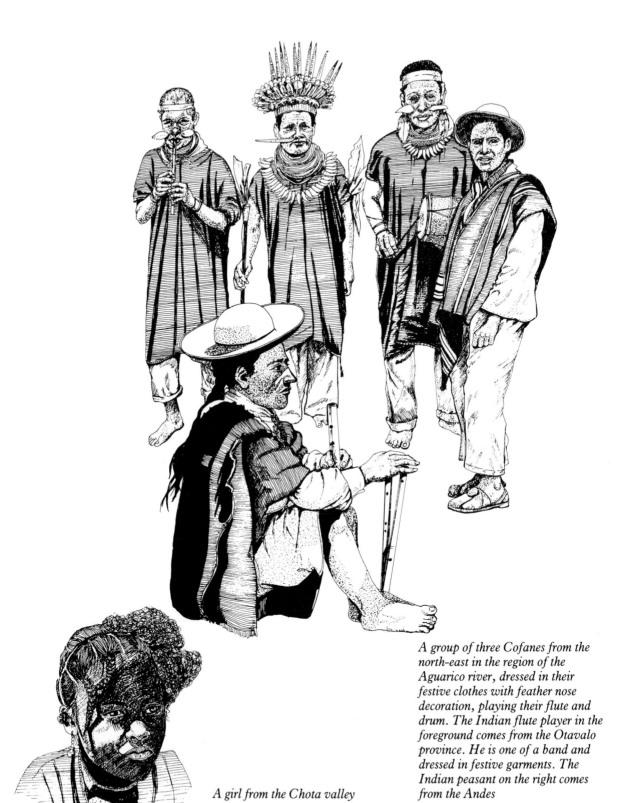

A group of three Cofanes from the north-east in the region of the Aguarico river, dressed in their festive clothes with feather nose decoration, playing their flute and drum. The Indian flute player in the foreground comes from the Otavalo province. He is one of a band and dressed in festive garments. The Indian peasant on the right comes from the Andes

A girl from the Chota valley

GUYANA

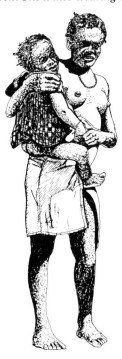

This typical girl from Guyana who works in the fields, carries her load on her back suspended by a broad band over her head. This is the traditional way of also carrying their children. She is also wearing a queyu

Woman wearing a queyu, carrying her baby

Guyana is an Amerindian word meaning 'land of waters'. The country is about the size of Britain yet a very small percentage of the land is cultivated. More than three quarters of the country consists of an almost impenetrable jungle and forest region which runs down from the upland savanna of the Rupununi and Kanaku mountains. Most of the population live in a narrow strip of the country, never more than 5 kilometres deep, which runs along the coast. Most of Guyana's agricultural land is in this narrow strip, agriculture only being possible by a complicated system of dykes and drains.

Agriculture is largely in the hands of Guyanese of East Indian descent, families who migrated to Guyana from India as indentured labour in the nineteenth century. Africans, originally brought to Guyana as slaves from the seventeeth to the nineteenth centuries, have tended to shun agriculture for urban occupations. The population, of about 810 thousand consists of 1% European, 61% East Indian, 32% African, the remaining 6% made up of Chinese, Portugese, and indigenous Indians. A quarter of the population lives in the capital, Georgetown.

The Amerindians of Guyana belong to the Arawak and Carib groups and are rapidly being brought into contact with the rest of society as a result of government policies and the economic penetration of the areas in which they live. Although less numerous than the East Indians, power is held by the African group in Guyana. It is the only English speaking country in South America.

Amongst the Caribs it is customary to wear a wide knitted cotton band around the ankles and just below the knees, the tightness of which causes the calf muscles to swell abnormally. occasionally the arms are also thus treated. The Macusi and the Arecuna tribes use a similar band to constrict their ankles.

Some tribes, especially the Carib women, pierce one or more holes in their lower lips through which they pass a pin or piece of pointed wood. Similarly, the men pierce a hole just under the

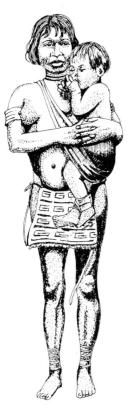

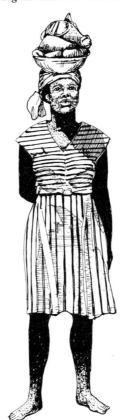

Girl at the Paramaribo market carrying her wares on her head

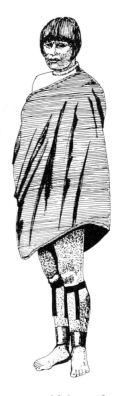

Macusi woman carrying her baby in a sling. She wears a band of cotton just above the ankles and upper arms. She is wearing a small apron called a queyu

Carib woman with just a shawl around her. She has bands just above the ankle and below her knees

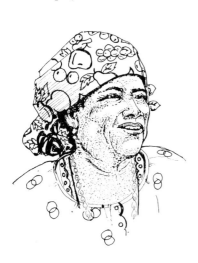

Woman wearing a typical headscarf

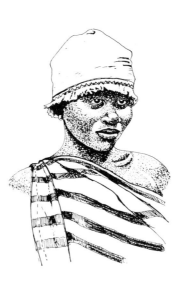

Creole schoolgirl

Tattoos on lips and chin, many wore obias *which are ankle rings against the evil spirits*

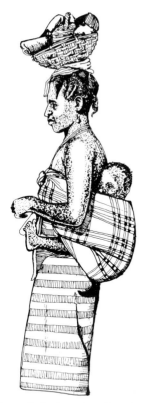

Carrying a baby in a shawl on the back and the shopping on the head

middle of their lower lip through which a loop of string is fastened inside the mouth. To this is attached a bell-shaped ornament made of shell or bone, with red and white streamers hanging down to the chin. They also pierce their noses in order to suspend a crescent-shaped ornament of highly polished copper or silver. The men, and sometimes even the women, also pierce their ears through which to stick pieces of straw.

The Indian men generally wear a piece of cloth known as a *lap*, hung from a cord tied around the waist. This used to be made of the inner bark of a tree, beaten until it became the texture of rough cloth. Nowadays it is made of a cotton material. The women wear a small square apron, known as a *queyu*, originally made of threaded seeds but, with the advent of traders, the seeds were replaced by coloured beadwork, both elaborate and artistic, the designs varying in different areas.

Occasionally, sandals are worn. These are made from the leaf stalk of a palm and held on with string that passed between the big toe and the next toe. As they are worn mainly on stoney ground they do not last long, but new ones can be made very quickly from the nearest leaf. The Indians' simplest mode of adornment is by painting the body, mainly for festive occasions. Tattooing is limited to a small distinctive tribal mark either on the arms or at the corner of the mouth.

Paint is applied with the use of several pigments, red and blue-black being the most popular colours. A man may paint both feet to the ankles in red, and completely cover his trunk in either blue-black or with an intricate pattern of lines. His face may be streaked red across the brige of the nose, with the two red lines in place of eyebrows, as well as on the forehead, and possibly spots and lines on the remainder of the face. Women have a broad band of blue-black painted from the corners of the mouth to the ears.

Necklaces made of bush-hogs' teeth are worn as a sign of hunting successes. On special occasions men also wear strings of seeds or beads around their wrists and ankles. They also smooth down their hair making it shiny with palm oil and parting it in the centre, daubing on masses of red paint on which to stick down white feathers. A long straw or stick decorated with feathers is worn through the lobe of each ear so that one end rested on the cheek, almost to the mouth.

Feather crowns are worn, the colour and shape varying with the tribes, with long strings hanging down the back to which are attached numerous tinkling items.

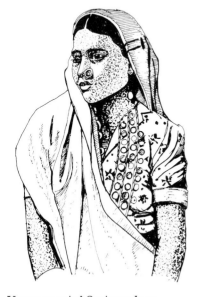

Young married Surinam-born Hindustani woman in full dress

Around the waist a plaited palm leaf skirt may be worn, and ruffs made of long tail feathers from local birds are fastened to the shoulders to stand at right angles to the body.

Women's attire is much simpler. They wear very few feathers, but masses of seeds and beads around their necks, waists, ankles, wrists and upper arms.

Macusi mothers carry their babies in front of them in a sling fastened over the right shoulder, but any other loads they carry on their backs suspended by a broad band over their foreheads.

Of the dancers in the interior, most of the girls smear their legs from knee to ankle with white pipe clay dots. Around their ankles they wear *joro-joros* made of fibrous plaits with hard shells attached and accentuate the strict rhythm of the drum and shakers. The tall drums are held between the knees and beaten with both hands. The shakers are of calabash shells filled with hard dried fruit stones. Another simple percussion instrument consists of just a board and big drumsticks made of a hard wood.

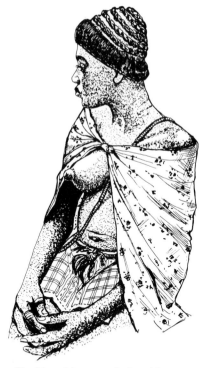

Fashionable young lady with a complicated hairstyle

Kondre Masra, the strong man ▶

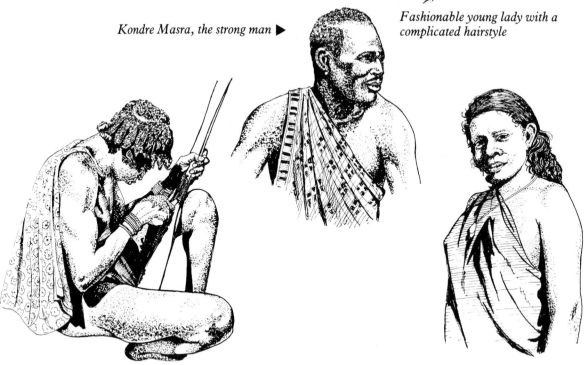

A Creole carving wood with a small knife

Carib Indian girl

44

PARAGUAY

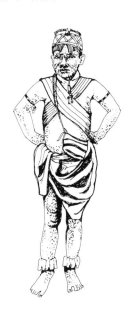

Lengua woman wearing a blanket, her only garment, worn like a kilt around her waist

Paraguay is the least well-known, most isolated country in South America despite its position in the centre of the continent. Paraguay is a country (like Bolivia) completely landlocked bordered by Argentina, Bolivia, and Brazil all of whom, in different ways, have exerted an influence. The River Paraguay cuts the country into two distinct parts; the Paraná Plateau and the Chaco.

The Paraná Plateau region consists of a fertile plain, broken up by rolling wooded hills. The bulk of Paraguay's 3 million population live in this hilly region. The plains are given over to the production of agricultural goods; rice, tobacco, sugar, cereals, and cotton.

The Chaco, lying to the west of the Paraguay River is forest and pasture land. Close to the river are areas of grass and palm but further westwards the land becomes increasingly dry and bleak. The north west is virtually without water. The Chaco as a whole has few settlements apart from some Mennonite farmers and small settlements close to the river. Some 50 thousand Indian people – the Guayanas, Cainguas, and Guayakis – live peaceful lives in this region whose cultures are closer to the stone age than to the twentieth century.

The pre-columbian society of Paraguay consisted of the Guarani Indians, peaceful people who did not oppose the Spanish invasion of their culture. Spanish missionaries for over 150 years from the start of the seventeenth century established settlements, called *reductions*, in which Guarani Indians were encouraged to settle and learn skills. They built magnificent churches utilizing their new-found skills as carpenters, masons, and painters. After the Jesuit missionaries were expelled in 1767 the settlements disintegrated, the Indians were made serfs by new masters, the churches fell into disrepair or were destroyed. A few still remain in Paraguay.

Immigration into Paraguay has not been as marked as elsewhere on the continent, although some 25% of Paraguayans live abroad for economic or polical reasons. The majority of

Toba Indian boy of the Gran Chaco. He is dressed for a festival, the usual wear being just paint and feathers

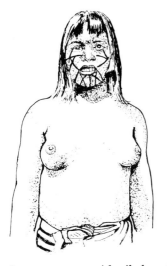

Lengua woman with tribal markings on her face. Her skin is a reddish brown

Guaycuru Indian of the Gran Chaco in a jaguar skin helmet and tooth necklace

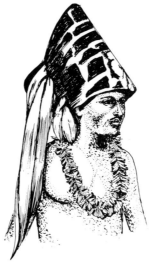

Woman working on a tobacco plantation with a typical head covering ▶

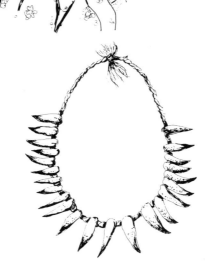

The bride of a rural wedding

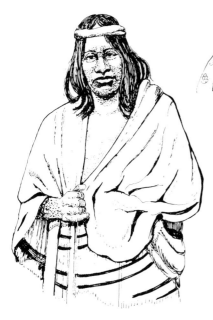

Lengua Indian wrapped in a blanket-like garment made of fine wool

Necklace made of jaguar teeth

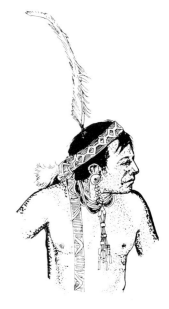

Native Indian dancer with a feathered headdress

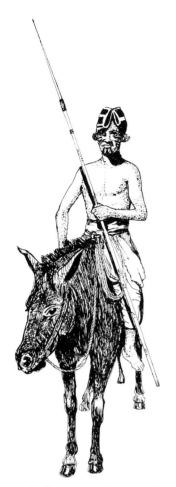

Paraguayans are of mixed Spanish and Guarani blood. The Guarani language has survived to the extent that it is the second language to Spanish.

Paraguay lies across the Tropic of Capricorn and its name is thought to be either a corruption of *Payagua*, the name of an Indian tribe, or *Paraguari* meaning palmcrown.

Cattle farming forms a vast part of the industry, the ranch workers, equipped with lassos and bolas, wear ponchos which can also act as waterproof overcoats or blankets.

One of the characteristics of the Guaycuru Indians of the Gran Chaco is the wearing of a jaguar skin helmet, signifying their great hunting prowess. Some camouflage themselves with creepers when hunting birds such as ostriches which are considered a delicacy, apart from the value of their feathers.

The Toba Indians also of the Gran Chaco mainly wear paint and feathers in preference to clothing. The Lengua Indians, whose faces are often disfigured by tribal marks, are noted for their pure wool distinctive patterned blankets. The men fasten these around their waists like a kilt. Each district has its own design. The colours black and white are from natural wool, red is made from the cochineal insect, whilst yellows and browns are prepared from various tree barks. These blankets are woven and spun in fine texture by the women.

Lengua Indian mounted on a mule carrying a large spear for fishing. He is wearing a traditional woollen cap and his face is adorned with tribal markings

A bolas, which is a throwing weapon ▶ made of balls attached to cords, used mainly for hunting large game and cattle

A horseman with the skin of a jaguar ▶▶ he has just killed slung over his horse. He is carrying bolas

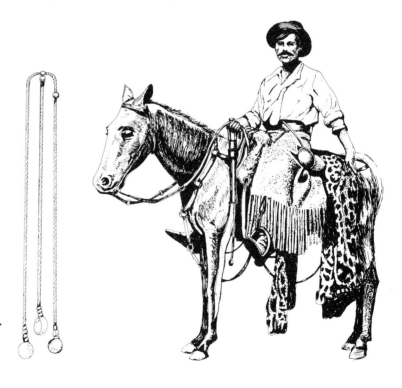

47

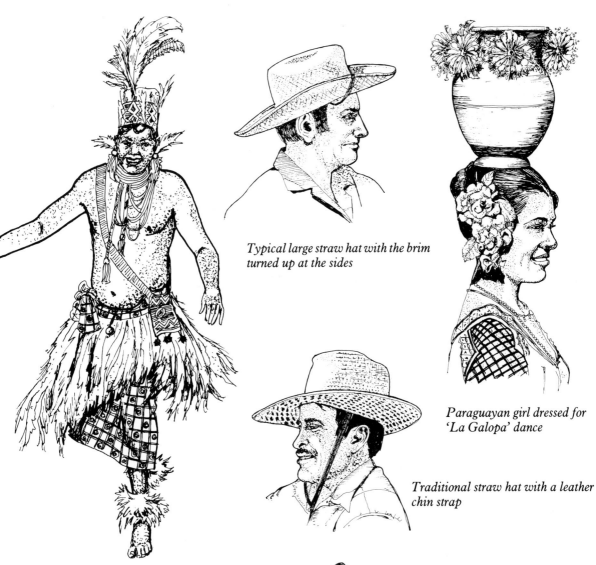

Typical large straw hat with the brim turned up at the sides

Paraguayan girl dressed for 'La Galopa' dance

Traditional straw hat with a leather chin strap

Dressed in feathers with a red and white skirt, hat and shoulder bag for a native dance

Dancers of 'La Chiperita'. The man ▶ would wear a black and white patterned shirt, black trousers, and a red and black striped poncho; the girl a black blouse with white lace sleeves and trimmings and the white shirt with a colourful border at the base

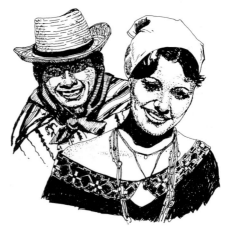

PERU

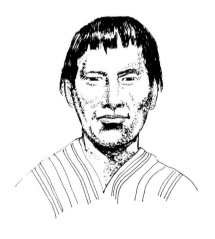

Peruvian Indian wearing a traditional headdress. The flat hat has a narrow turned-up brim worn over a knitted helmet or chullo. These hats can be in varying designs. The waist length hair is beaded and plaited with tassels at the ends

Typical Quechua Indian boy with a fringed hairstyle

Geography has played a major part in shaping the history of South America. Nowhere on the continent is this more true than in Peru. The third largest country in South America, more than twice the size of France, Peru is divided into three distinct regions. The coast region, a long strip of desert with little rainfall, represents 11% of the country yet absorbs 44% of the nearly 19 million population. Agriculture thrives in this region thanks to irrigation; fishing is an important coastal industry. Lima, the capital city, dominates the coastal area.

The Sierra, the Andean mountain ranges, are the location of Peru's mining industry a region shared with large numbers of Indian people involved in subsistence agriculture and livestock raising. The Sierra covers 26% of the area of Peru in which half of the population live. The Montaña, or Selva, the eastern half of the Andes together with an area of jungle and tropical rain forests accounts for 62% of Peru's area yet contains just 5% of the population. In recent years the Montaña has enjoyed a boom from rubber, the growing of coca leaves, and the cultivation of sugar, coffee, and fruit for the Lima market. Each distinct region of Peru has its own character and economy.

Peru was the centre of the Inca empire which spread throughout South America. The Indian population living in the Sierra are the Inca's descendants. Between 30- and 40% of Peru's population are Quechua- and Aymara-speaking Indians most of whom live in traditional communities outside a money economy and the rest of society. Their educational level is minimal; health, and living conditions poor. Yet the culture they have inherited from the Incas is a rich one that gives a shape to their lives. About a tenth of Peruvian society is white, descended from the Spanish. Apart from a small number of Black and Asian people the rest of Peruvian society consists of Cholos, as the *mestizos* of Peru are known.

Throughout the colonial period Peru was an important source of silver to Spain. Astronomical wealth came from the mines of Potosi (now in Bolivia) and the rich veins in the

49

Peruvian Sierra. Lima became known as the 'City of Kings'; the Spanish culture was indelibly stamped upon the whole of Peru. Indian revolts against Spain preceded Peru's independence in 1821. Independence failed to bring either prosperity or stability to Peru, especially not to the Indian people whose lot worsened.

The extent of guano gave Peru a boom in the early nineteenth century after which, fortunately, Peru has been able to produce a variety of exports. With the development of new industries and new agricultural products Peru became increasingly urbanised throughout the twentieth century though always her geography maintained the distinctive shape, and ordered the progress of, the country.

The people of Peru vary from the sophisticated living in the coastal region to the primitive tribes living in the remote jungle. Between these extremes every variety is to be found.

The Sierra or mountainous area has settlements mainly of Quechua Indians. The Quechua and Aymará Indians at one time were predominant in the Andean uplands, but gradually the Inca Empire went into decline, accelerated by the Spanish occupation. The characteristics of the mountain Indians of Peru are similar to those of the Bolivian Indians, each having their own *chacara* or land where they grow all the food they need. Their requirements in clothing are very simple, consisting of rough hand-woven garments: the inevitable poncho, and a locally-made felt or straw hat with a large turned up brim with a close fitting woollen cap beneath, also short warm trousers with white underpants. The backs of the trousers are slashed – a variable length and style for different villages – to show more or less of the underpants. A pair of raw hide sandals and a fabric saddle-bag may be hung over the shoulder and would complete their needs.

There is little variety in their clothing, many of the tribes wearing almost nothing except in the districts where mosquitoes abound, and in such areas a long shirt known as a *cushma* is worn, made of a cotton fibre that is woven by the women.

In the Putumayo region, clothing is dispensed with entirely, pigments of red, yellow and white, being smeared on the skin instead.

Cuzco, capital of the Inca Empire, is still inhabited by Quechua Indians. They wear bright costumes reminiscent of the Spanish bull-ring. The Quechua women spin the native cloth of Peru from the llama and alpaca to make heavy woollen shawls. They wear thick petticoats and skirts. The most

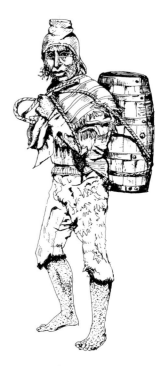

The Inca Indians in Cuzco peddle water from a barrel roped to their backs wearing clothes that are in shreds. They are a disappearing type

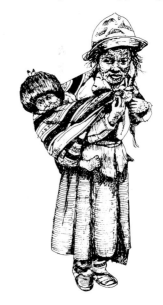

Chola girl carrying a baby on her back in a shawl in the traditional way

50

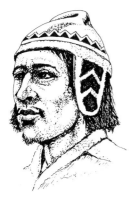

Peruvian Quechua Indian wearing a cap with earflaps

distinctive feature of their appearance is a reversible pancake hat made of straw. One side is covered with gaudy tinsel, and the other with a coarse woollen material, almost waterproof. To distinguish the tribes from one another, various tassels and fringes are displayed on both sides of the headdress. The Quechua often use silver spoons as hair ornamentation.

There are some hundred Indian tribes living in the jungle of Eastern Peru in complete isolation, speaking their own languages and living in very primitive conditions.

Another section are the descendants of the Quechua and Aymará Indians, most of whom live in the highlands of the Andes. They cling tenaceously to their traditional culture, and after four centuries of European culture they have accepted very little.

Most Peruvian Indian tribes make ▶ simple musical pipes from hollow reeds with three holes at the lower end that emit thin and melancholy notes

◀ An Indian in traditional dress. The trousers are three-quarter length. The open shirt and sleeveless jacket are covered by a poncho

In the valley of the Pangoa river the Indians belong to many subdivisions of the Campa tribe. They wear sleeveless gowns, being keen hunters with bow and arrow, and plumed crowns and garlands

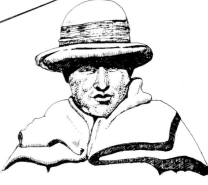

Quechuas are the original Indians of the Peruvian Sierra who formed the great population of the Inca dynasty. They wear mainly rough handspun and locally made straw or felt hats

51

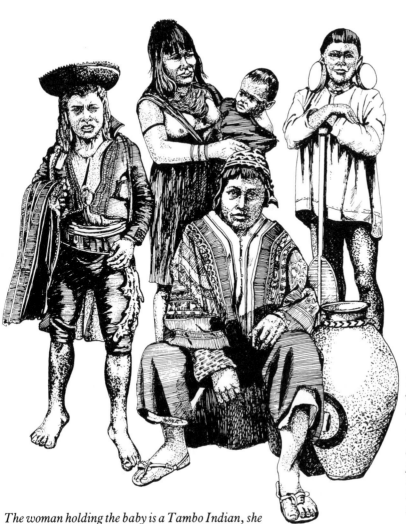

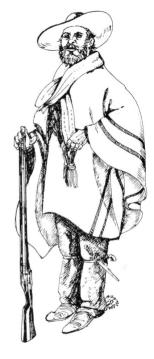

The costume of an ancient Inca warrier carrying a small halberd, the traditional weapon of the Incas

The travelling dress of the cordillera area. The hat is of felt, and the poncho and scarf of llama wool. The legwear is of vicuna leather with a knife worn in the kneeband. Large silver spurs were always popular

The woman holding the baby is a Tambo Indian, she is wearing masses of beads and a disc-shaped ornament from her nose. The other girl lives on the Napo river and is an Orejone, meaning big ears. This name was given to them as they wear immense wooden discs, thus enlarging their earlobes. The Indian on the left is dressed in a cloak, his outfit suggesting a bull ring. His hair is in ringlets. The seated Indian from the high plateau of Titicaca is wearing a brightly coloured poncho and a knitted cap with earflaps

Woman of the Campa, her face ▶ *decorated with tribal markings. The masses of beads were a sign of importance and wealth*

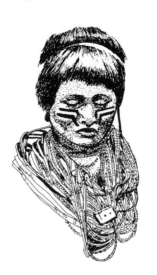

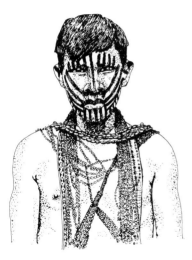

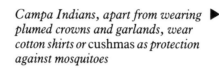

Campa Indians, apart from wearing plumed crowns and garlands, wear cotton shirts or cushmas as protection against mosquitoes ▶

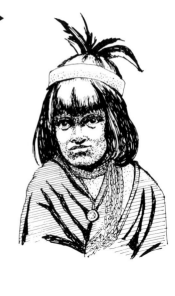

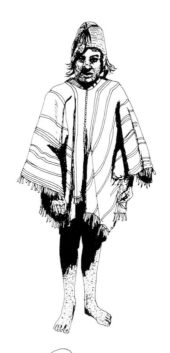

When a Peruvian travels he usually daubs his face with scarlet dye, indicating to which tribe he belongs. The seed and bead necklaces he wears are his only possessions

Cuzco, capital of the Inca Empire is ▶ still inhabited by Indians with Inca blood. This boy is wearing a woollen hat and poncho

Indian playing his flute, wearing a felt hat over a knitted cap. He has a shawl or serape over his shoulders which could be fringed. The most usual colours of these garments are ◀ reds, yellows, oranges and greens

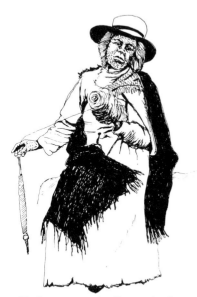

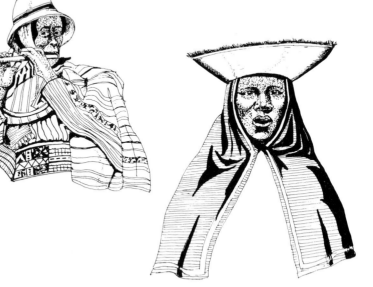

Chola women who live up in the mountains spin a coarse yarn from crude wool. This yarn is made up to produce almost all their clothing

Hat with a turned-up brim worn over a manta

URUGUAY

Although Uruguay is the smallest country in South America it is, nonetheless, a country the size of England and Wales combined. It's population, at 3 million, is less than that of Wales alone. Unlike other South American countries there is no great geographical diversity in Uruguay. The general appearance of the country is of gently undulating land, unbroken but for a few forested areas. A strip of plain edges the coast with flood plains in the west close to the border with Argentina. There are no great mountain ranges here, just gently sloping hills rising towards Brazil in the north. Argentina lies to the west, separated from Uruguay by the River Uruguay. The Atlantic coast is to the east, the estuary of the River Plate to the west. Uruguay's black soil is even richer than that of Argentina although little is used for arable farming. The economy, as it became under Spanish rule, is based predominantly upon cattle raising. Once they were introduced into Uruguay cattle rapidly multiplied feeding off her rich pastures. Gauchos, nomadic hunters, sought them for their hides living off their meat as they followed them around the country. This system gave way to a more commercial exploitation of cattle based upon large estates, the *estancias*, which, by the end of the nineteenth century, were providing meat and meat products to Europe. Wool, from the mid nineteenth century, became an important export.

There are no Indian people left in Uruguay, and few *mestizos*. Half the population lives in the capital, Montevideo, with a drift towards the towns continuing. The Roman Catholic Church was disestablished in 1919, all religious bodies now being equally tolerated.

The dress of the Charrua, a semi-nomadic hunting race originally from Entre Rios has changed little. They still wear garments of untanned hide and the typical headband and raw hide shoes. The shawl is woven on native looms and is worn draped around the waist along with the bolas.

The gaucho wears a loose fitting poncho and bombachos. His legs are covered with voluminous cotton or woollen pantaloons, gathered at the waist and ankles. When it is cold a chirpá or large woollen shawl is folded around the waist.

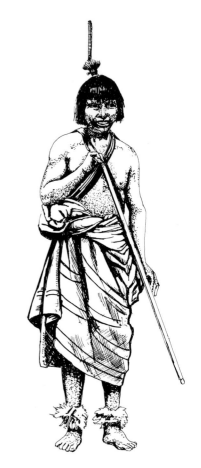

Charrua Indian in festive dress

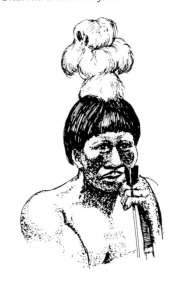

Charrua Indian with ceremonial headdress

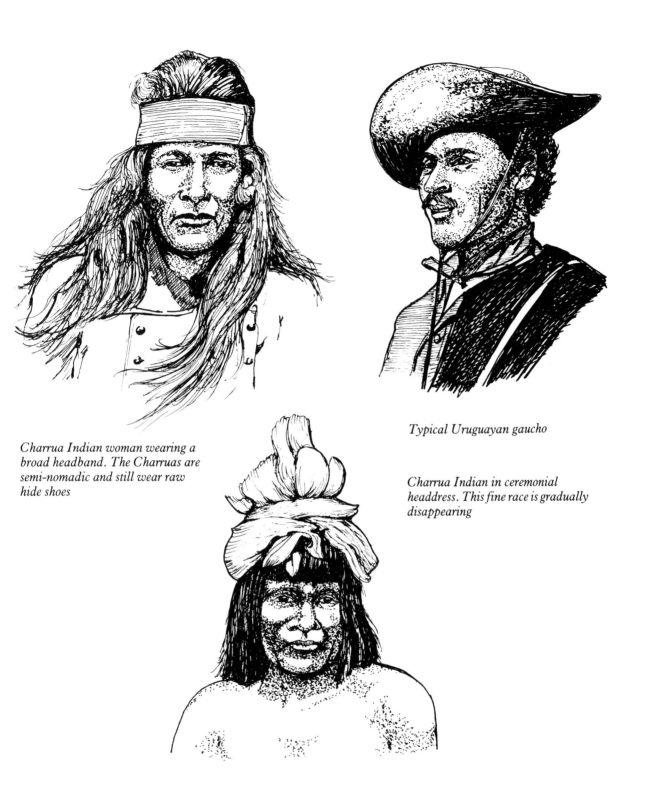

Typical Uruguayan gaucho

Charrua Indian woman wearing a broad headband. The Charruas are semi-nomadic and still wear raw hide shoes

Charrua Indian in ceremonial headdress. This fine race is gradually disappearing

VENEZUELA

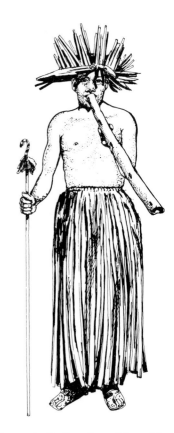

Taurepán Indian dressed in a skirt and hat, both of palm leaves

Venezuela was a backwater of the Spanish empire. There was little gold and silver to be found and, almost in desperation, the Spanish turned to agriculture. Venezuela was still a poor, agrarian society at the start of the twentieth century when oil was discovered which dramatically changed her fortunes. Venezuela is now the richest country in South America and one of the world's largest producers of oil.

Venezuela is the sixth largest country in South America with a population of 14 million which is small by comparison with other countries on the continent. Her long coastline on the Caribbean Sea stretches for 2,800 kilometres. To the east lies Guyana, to the south Brazil, and to the west Colombia. The country is usually divided geographically into four regions: the Venezuelan Highlands, part of the Andes chain, are in the west of the country and run along the coast; the Lowlands around the fresh-water lake of Maracaibo were transformed by the discovery of oil in 1914, and is one of the most prosperous areas of Venezuela; the vast central plain of the llanos of the River Orinoco where large herds of cattle and horses are reared; and the Guyana Highlands which account for half the country. Until recently the two latter regions were of little economic importance but are now important mineral producers where vast iron ore deposits are being mined, and from where 30% of Venezuela's oil now comes. Economic expansion has encroached upon the Indian people of Venezuela who live in the Guyanese Highlands, and in the forests west of Lake Maracaibo. Most of the population consists of *mestizos*, with a small African and Mulatto element along the coast. Immigration has been important in Venezuela since the Second World War shown by the fact that one in six of all Venezuelans was born abroad. Venezuela is a young society; over half the population are under 18 years. More than three quarters of Venezuelans live in cities and towns, and their dress is westernised.

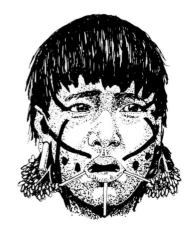

Indian face with tribal markings, rolled leaves through his earlobes, his mouth pierced with straws

Until 1829 when it became a separate Republic, Venezuela was part of the Republic of Colombia with Ecuador. Aboriginal inhabitants however still practise their traditional customs along the north-eastern frontier and in the Guyanan forests.

The Waiogomo Indians, a branch of the Caribs, are scattered in the dense forests as well as around the river. One of their tribal characteristics is their lack of dress. Short lengths of coarse material or aprons made of palm fibre are their everyday wear.

Until the mid twentieth century when American influence became apparent, Venezuelan culture was mainly Spanish and African in origin, the idigenous Indians contributing very little. The main folklore stems from the llanero.

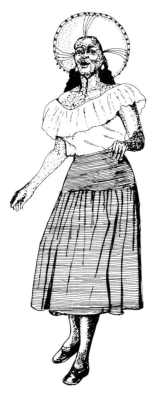

The woman is wearing a large straw hat with a turned up brim. The short sleeved blouse, usually of cotton, has a boat shaped neckline and is decorated with a deep frill

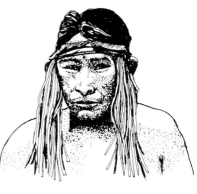

Chaké Indian wearing a typical ▶ *headdress*

Woman and child of the Maquiritare tribe. This nomadic tribe also live in the hinterland of Guyana. The absence of dress is one of their tribal characteristics

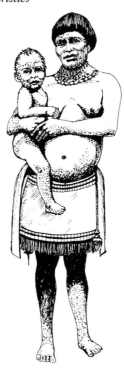

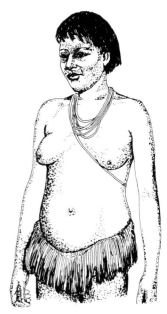

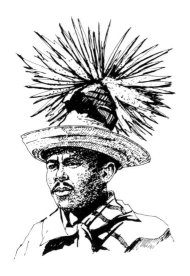

Straw hat with palm leaf decoration

Sanema Indian girl with a short fibre skirt

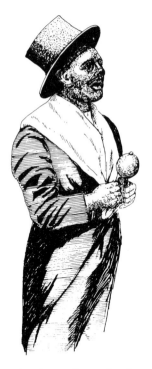

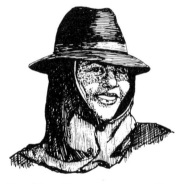

Traditional hat is a type of trilby worn over a hood and can be made of straw or felt

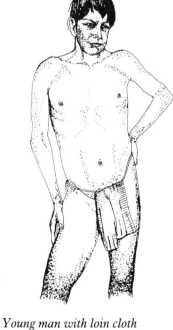

Top hat and morning dress, traditional of the Venezeulan Negro. He is holding a maraca

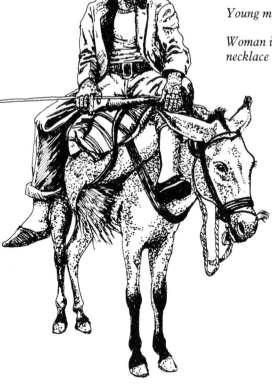

Young man with loin cloth

Woman in a loin cloth and a bead necklace

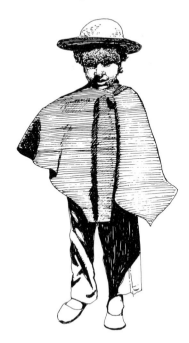

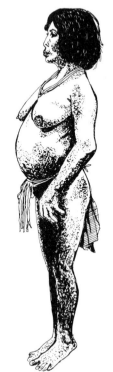

Small boy in a poncho and straw hat

The donkey, the chief pack animal is the common mode of travel in the mountains

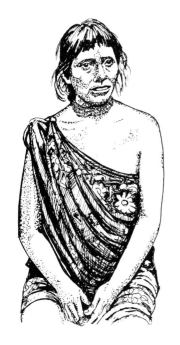

Typical dress of the Indian women who live on pile dwellings around Lake Maracaibo

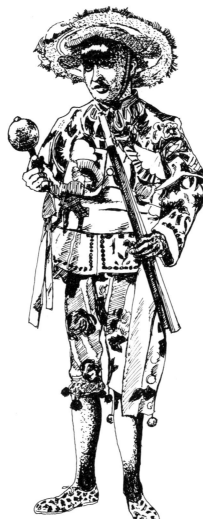

Dancer of the Candelaria

Waiomgomo Indian in his forest ▶ clothing of palm fibres. They also live in the Guyanan jungle

Indian of the Andes in a long poncho

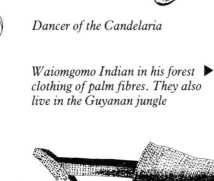

Woman wearing a soft straw hat

Indian sandal made in three parts

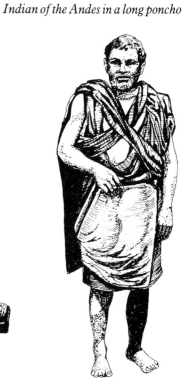

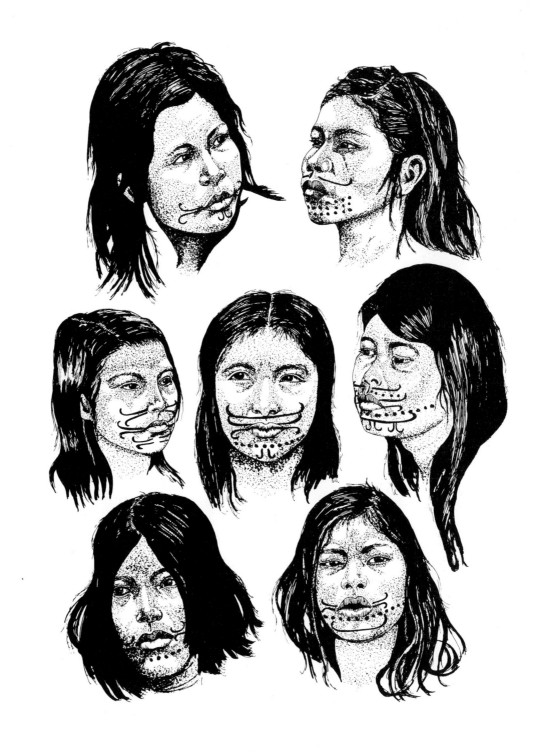

*Face paintings of Indian tribal markings used in
Colombia, Ecuador, Guyana and Venezuela*

GLOSSARY OF COSTUME TERMS

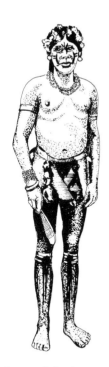

The knitted chullo *has beaded side pieces with tasselled ends and is worn by both men and women*

Wauwai man of the Amazon area painted and decorated with coloured string and beads. The face and legs have tribal markings, and the headdress is of flowers

Basque	A short skirt frill on a bodice
Bombachas	Long baggy trousers gathered at the ankles and held at the waist by a silver-studded leather belt. Worn by gauchos
Chamanto	A blanket worn between the legs like trousers and fastened with a belt
Chupalla	A woven straw hat worn by farm workers
Charahuilla	Very wide trousers tied at the ankles
Chirpá or chiripá	A square of coloured cloth which forms a kind of skirt worn over the gaucho's long baggy trousers (bombachas)
Chullo or llucho	Knitted or woven tight-fitting helmet
Chumbe	A white cloth belt decorated with coloured painting
Cushma	A long cotton shirt worn in Peru
Lap	A small piece of cotton cloth hung from a cord tied round the waist
Llucho or chullo	Knitted or woven tight-fitting helmet
Manto	A long narrow piece of black material draped over the head, around the face, and folded over and pinned at the neckline. A development of the Spanish mantilla
Mochila	Traditional native carrying bag
Obias	Ankle rings worn to ward off evil spirits
Paruma	Dress of chamba palm leaves worn by the Yagua Indians

Poncho	An oblong piece of woollen or alpaca cloth with a slit in the centre for the head to protrude, allowing the folds to cover the shoulders and arms to the elbows, and to fall down in front and behind
Queyu	Small square apron worn by women in Guyana
Ruana	Type of poncho
Serape	A type of shawl
Tupa	Breast ornament hung with silver coins
Yuburunasi	A type a bag slung over the back in which to carry a small baby

Open sandals, usually made of a rough hide

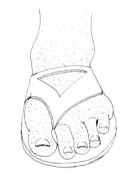

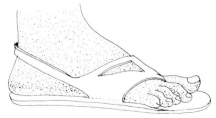

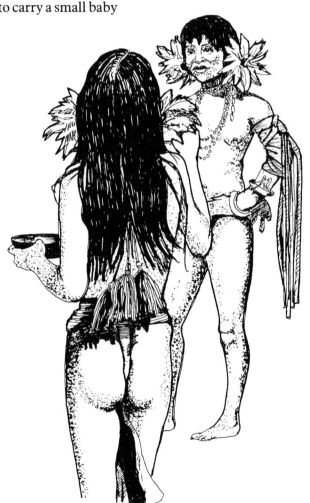

Young Karaja Indian girls from the Island of Bananal – Brazil

62

BIBLIOGRAPHY

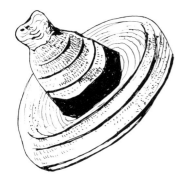

Sombrero of Cúpira

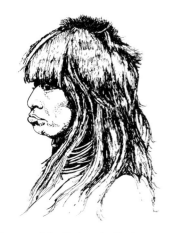

*Woman of the Pajonal tribe in Peru,
noted for their savagery in the past*

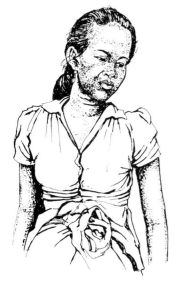

Surinam-born Javanese girl

ARETZ, ISABEL, *El Traje del Venezolano*, Monte Avila Editores,
  Venezuela 1976
ARTHAUD, C and HERBERT-STEVENS, F, *The Andes, Roof of
  America*, Vanguard Press 1956
BOUILLY, V, *Argentina Turistica*, Editions Delroisse, France 1977
BRUHN, W, and TILKE, M, *Pictorial History of Costume*, Zwemmer
  1955
BUSTAMANTE, EDGAR, *Maravilloso Ecuador*, Circulo de Lectores,
  S A Quito, Ecuador 1978
CLARKE, MARREBE, *Bolivia – Country and People*, Oxfam Education
  1979
CUEVA, JUAN, *Equador*, Editions Delroisse, France
EDWARDS, AUGUSTIN, *Peoples of Old*, Benn 1929
GILBERT, JOHN, *National Costumes of the World*, Hamlyn 1972
GRIFFITHS, JOHN, *Let's Visit Bolivia*, Burke Publishing 1984
HAMMERTON, J A, *Lands and Peoples*, Amalgamated Press, 1927
HAMMERTON, J A, *People of all Nations*, Amalgamated Press
  1922-1924
HARROLD, R, *Folk Costumes of the World*, Blandford Press 1978
HUXLEY, MATTHEW, and CAPA, CORNELL, *Farewell to Eden*, Chatto
  and Windus 1965
KARFELD, K P, *Brazil*, Brazilian Foreign Office 1972
LUZUY, P, and BOUTANG, P A, *Faces of Bronze*, The Oldbourne
  Press, London
LYLE, G, and CALDWELL, J C, *Let's visit Argentina*, Burke
  Publishing 1983
MANN, H, *South America*, Thames and Hudson 1957
MANSON, JEAN, ASTURRAS, MIGUEL-ANGEL and DIEZ DE
  MEDINA, F, *Bolivia, an Undiscovered Land*, Harrap 1961
MOREL, G P, editor, *Revista Chile*, Cultural Affairs and
  Information Directorate of the Chilean Ministry for Foreign
  Affairs 1979
ROITER, FULVOIR, *Brazil*, Atlantis Verlag, Zurich 1969 and
  Thames Hudson 1971
SAFI, JULIAN, *Uruguay*, Editions Delroisse, France
SUMWALT, M M, *Colombia in Pictures*, The Oak Tree Press 1968
VAN DEL POLL, W, *Surinam, The Country and its People*, W van
  Hoeve, The Hague 1951
Tipos e Aspectos du Brazil, Coletanea de Illustracoes Publicados na
  Revista Brasileira de Geografia 1944
Paraguay, Editions Delroisse, France
THORN, E F, *Among the Indians of Guiana*, Kegan Paul 1883
TURNER-WILCOX, R, *Folk and Festival Costumes of the World*,
  Batsford 1965